DR. CASS INGRAM'S

Natural Cures *for* Headaches

D1297645

Knowledge House
Buffalo Grove, Illinois

Printed in the United States of America
First Edition

This book contains information, advice and observations related to the study of migraines and other headaches. This book is not intended as a substitute for medical diagnosis or treatment. The reader who has a serious disease should consult a physician before initiating any change in his/her treatment or before beginning any new treatment.

ISBN: 1-931078-09-2

For ordering information call: 1-800-243-5242

For email inquires: www.headachecure@p-73.com

Contents

DEDICATION

For those who are suffering and wish to suffer no longer.

Introduction

Migraine headaches are one of the major plagues of modern civilization. Millions of people all over the world are afflicted with this dreaded illness. However, migraines, as well as the majority of other types of headaches, are more common in the USA than anywhere else in the world. The fact is in North America chronic headaches are truly an unmerciful plague.

Though migraine headaches are among the most common of all ailments afflicting modern man, they are not a new disease. Rather, they have existed for thousands of years. The ancient Egyptians and Greeks experienced them. Then, no one knew the cause. Yet, the ancients did ponder over the possibility that food reactions were partly to blame. Just what caused the pain of migraine remained an enigma until 1913, when two Frenchmen, Doctors Lesne and Richet, proposed that food allergy was the likely culprit. Unfortunately, few took note of their observation. To this day the cause of migraines continues to remain unknown to most medical researchers and practitioners.

In the past, treatments for migraines have been crude and ineffective. Everything from surgery to herbs and poultices have been tried, to no avail. The reason these treatments failed was that they neglected to address the cause. The sufferers of old found little or no relief for their migraines. They didn't even have painkilling drugs. Yet, the situation is little better today. Except for drugs, modern "migraineurs" find little or no hope in the orthodox medical profession for relief or cure.

This is why various alternative treatments are pursued. These treatments include acupuncture, chiropractic, nutritional therapy, homeopathy, osteopathy, biofeedback, physical therapy, massage, and even faith healing. This is because one thing is universal: they must continue on with the hope of finding a cure, as their pain is often so agonizing that they wish to die.

It is understandable that headache victims feel this way. Yet, they should never lose hope for a cure. They need not continue suffering from severe headaches for untold numbers of years. This is because there are answers. Many of these answers are found in modest lifestyle changes. Others are various natural medicines, which halt headache pain. Still others are certain structural therapies which remove the cause of headaches.

In respect to chronic illnesses modern medicine offers few if any cures. In regard to migraines physicians rely primarily upon drugs which are impotent in achieving long-term cures. Medications may be used to abort certain types of headaches and are often useful for relieving the pain. Yet, even the most potent medications often fail to curb headache pain. Plus, there is always the risk of side effects.

Today, migraine has become its own unique disease. Up to 20% of the population is affected. Thus, there are literally millions of sufferers. What's more, each person has developed his/her own unique migraine pattern. Some suffer from migraines on a monthly basis, others weekly, and some unfortunate souls have them every day. Since there are many kinds of headaches the question might arise: Exactly what constitutes a migraine? This subject will be addressed in the forthcoming chapters.

In the United States headaches cause a greater degree of pain for a greater number of people than any other single condition. Every day approximately 13 million Americans suffer from headaches, and a large percentage of these are migraines. Most of these sufferers have the impression that their headaches are largely incurable. They know no other options besides medication and bed rest; they are told that nothing else can be done. The fact is there are a number of answers far superior in curative potential than medication and bed rest. Are these answers biofeedback, stress reduction, and psychoanalysis? Not in the least. To cure migraines is to understand them and to uncover the underlying cause. None of the "mental" or anti-stress therapies even begin to approach the cause, at least in the majority of instances. In fact, stress as a primary cause of headaches is exceedingly rare.

If stress and emotional problems are not the primary cause, what is the missing factor? Many people overlook the fact that the vast majority of migraine headaches result from physical problems, physical derangements, and physical diseases, not mental or psychological ones.

This book makes one simple claim. It is that migraine headaches can be cured *if* the cause is discovered and *if* appropriate treatment is prescribed. In the majority of instances that cause is food allergies. Certainly, these are strong words. Yet, these statements are based upon years of clinical experience and a plethora of scientific data. Plus, this makes a great deal of sense, and common sense is important in the author's view and in the view of many patients as well. In other words, diet is a major factor in a variety of diseases and migraines are no exception.

Let it be reiterated that migraine headaches are a curable condition. The sufferer need not live with the pain. Why the repetition? Because most people feel that there are few options to pursue and that they have little choice other than to endure it. Medical doctors often proclaim that the most which can be done is to treat the symptoms in order to ease the pain. Nearly everyone knows that the primary treatment for migraines is over-the-counter medicine, such as aspirin and Tylenol, and millions of dollars of these are sold each month. In severe cases mood-altering drugs, such as Cafergot, Inderal, Midrin, Prozac, Xanax, and Valium, are prescribed. Some pain-ridden individuals are given injections of potent narcotics, like Demerol and Percocet, to gain relief. This is a common prescription in emergency rooms.

In regard to the diagnosis and treatment of migraines it is important to keep an open mind. The current medical model for treatment is inadequate. The exceptions are those migraines which are due to serious, underlying disease.

There is little scientific proof that medicines aid in the elimination of headaches. Rather, they serve only to treat the symptoms. Aspirin is an excellent example. Americans consume over 70 billion tablets of aspirin every year, which amounts to a staggering 20 million pills per day. Headache is the number one illness for which aspirin is used. Arthritis is next, with back pain and fever also resulting in significant consumption. Through all this aspirin usage is the incidence of migraine or arthritis decreasing? No—both diseases are on the rise.

Incredibly, there are people who take aspirin, even though they have no aches or pains. Every day they take it on the supposition that an aspirin a day will keep the doctor away, that is, the cardiovascular surgeon or cardiologist. This is because aspirin thins the blood and may slightly decrease the risk of heart attack and stroke. However, new research indicates that risks for digestive disorders, internal bleeding—including life-threatening intracranial bleeding—and cancer are significantly increased as a result of daily aspirin intake. Studies even show that it causes cancer of the internal organs. In particular, the pancreas is highly vulnerable to its toxic effects. Women who regularly take aspirin have a much higher risk for pancreatic cancer than the norm.

Aspirin is not candy. Unfortunately, some children think so. Far from innocuous, it accounts for more cases of childhood illness and death than any other pill or poison. Plus, it is responsible for the fatal childhood disease known as *Reye's Syndrome*. Thus, aspirin is a deadly poison. It should never be given to children. Why play with fire?

Each year, thousands of people become ill and hundreds die as a result of aspirin toxicity. The author knows personally of patients who consumed 10 to 20 or more aspirin per day, often for several days continuously, in an attempt to relieve headache pain. Many who consumed such massive doses suffer physiological damage to this day. In high doses aspirin damages tissues throughout the body, including the lining of the stomach and intestines, the liver, arteries, veins, brain, and kidneys. Regular aspirin intake leads to the depletion of a wide range of nutrients, including vitamin C, vitamin K, folic acid, vitamin B12, magnesium, calcium, and zinc. The immune system is negatively affected. Certain adult aspirin users can develop a Reye's-like syndrome involving chronic viral infections—not enough to kill, but enough to debilitate. As a result of regular aspirin intake such individuals are highly vulnerable to recurrent viral infections as well as to infections by yeasts and parasites. It becomes clear that aspirin has a negative effect on virtually all body systems. It impairs immunity, damages the intestines, irritates the liver, and inflames the kidneys. By all this aspirin-induced trauma the susceptibility to migraines actually increases. In the extreme Reye's syndrome can develop, which is a viral infection of the brain occurring in children. It is usually fatal.

It is understandable that drugs may be taken to ease the pain. However, this is a temporary measure. Of greater significance is to eradicate the problem altogether. Nothing can be more important than that. The primary goal of any reasonable treatment plan would be to eliminate the headaches forever. At a minimum the headaches should be reduced in frequency and severity. What could be more important than to be free, finally, of all the pain, agony, irritability, frustration, and all the rest of the sickening feelings? Whatever the symptoms might be, if the cause is treated, they can all disappear.

What choice does the sufferer have, anyway? He/she must pursue any angle possible and cannot afford to be closed minded. Such an individual has already tried the orthodox medical approach. Often, hopes for a cure are dashed by comments such as, "There is no cure for migraine. You'll have to learn to live with it." The desperate patient presses the doctor to check more thoroughly, to try again to find a cause. The doctor will, albeit often reluctantly, run a battery of tests. The patient may be hospitalized to perform the tests, which often include sophisticated procedures such as CAT scans, MRIs, brain scans, angiographs, and other X-rays. Blood and urine tests are also performed. The hopeful patient awaits the verdict, but, invariably, the response is, "We checked everything, but all the tests are negative." Oh, what despair the patient must feel at that trying moment—the futility of it all: all that time, hope, and money in search for a cure, all for naught. Yet, frequently, all the patient was hoping for was an answer, any answer. These patients are willing to accept virtually any verdict—even that of a brain tumor—just to find out once and for all *why all the pain.* Ultimately, the migraine sufferer loses hope and slumps into the continuation of a seemingly endless nightmare—living with excruciating, mind-boggling, and sometimes mind-damaging pain.

Can migraines be serious? Can they kill? There is no question that some headaches are caused by life-threatening diseases such as brain tumors, meningitis, blood clots, and aneurysms. However, in terms of chronic migraine headaches these illnesses account for a very small minority. Fortunately, most people reading this book have had the more serious causes of headaches ruled out long ago. All that remains is a world of pain without any answers. For that majority this book provides information which, if applied, will change lives forever. It can give the reader a chance to be free of headache pain—permanently.

Chapter 1

What Started All This Pain?

Are you reading this book because you have migraines? If so, was a diagnosis ultimately made? Or, do you just know from the symptoms you experience? In most instances, those who know they have migraines have had the diagnosis confirmed by a physician. Usually, the patterns exhibited by the headache—the distribution of the pain, one side or both, the prodroma, a medical word for the symptoms occurring just prior to the headache's onset, and concurrent symptoms, such as nausea, vomiting, visual disturbances, etc. were all considered before the final diagnosis was made.

Even so, many important questions remain. Just what causes the headaches? Or, are there several causes to consider? When did they first begin? How long have they existed? How often do they occur? What precipitates them? How long do they last? What makes them worse? What gives them relief? Is there a history of a serious fall or accident? What is the dental history? Is there a family history of migraine and/or food allergy? Is there any history of serious disease or hospitalization? All these questions must be answered before an accurate assessment can be made and an appropriate treatment prescribed.

The history tells all regarding the underlying causes of migraines as well as other kinds of headaches. Unless a physician conducts a thorough history, as well as physical exam, potential causes will be missed. Such questions are the basis for a thorough history. Additional questions which are important to discern in the initial history include:

1. Is there a history of a whiplash or other traumatic injury occurring prior to the onset of the migraines?

2. Is there a long-term history of lower back trouble?

3. Is there a habit of sleeping on the stomach?

4. Does the patient often awaken with a headache?

5. Prior to a headache, does noticeable weight gain or swelling in the extremities occur?

6. If female, is there a history of premenstrual syndrome (PMS)?

7. Are depression, hair loss, and/or cold extremities coinciding symptoms?

8. Is there a history of symptoms associated with blood sugar disturbances, including irritability, fatigue, mood swings, falling asleep after meals, hyperactivity, mental confusion, depression, anxiety, agitation, and digestive disturbances?

9. Is there a history of chronic constipation?

10. Is the patient currently taking blood thinners, blood pressure medicines, and/or medications for heart disease?

11. Is there a history of high blood pressure?

12. Is there a history of severe, debilitating viral infections, particularly viral infections of the brain (encephalitis)?

13. Is there a history of lumbar puncture (spinal tap) for surgery or childbirth?

14. Is there a history of repeated traumatic car or motorcycle accidents?

15. Is there a history of traumatic falls on the head or on the buttocks (i.e. broken coccyx)?

There appears to be some confusion concerning how to classify the severity of migraines. Part of this is due to the bizarre frequency patterns which many headache sufferers experience. There are those whose headaches occur every day. Others experience weekly headaches. Some individuals have headaches that occur routinely every weekend. Still others have monthly or bimonthly headaches. Then again, the severity of these headaches differs with each case. For these reasons a unique evaluation method called the Migraine Intensity Exam has been devised. Take this test to evaluate the severity of your headaches.

Migraine Intensity Exam

Which of the following do you experience in regard to migraines either prior to or during the headache?

Points

1. The frequency is best described as:

    a) daily 30
    b) every other day 20
    c) twice per week 15
    d) once per week 10
    e) once per month 5

2. Pain resistant to medication .10

3. Swelling of the extremities, bloating, and/or weight gain . . .10

4. Bloodshot eyes 5

5. Nausea 5

6. Vomiting 10

7. Other digestive disturbances (diarrhea, constipation, stomach pain, etc.) 5

8. Sensitivity to light or sound 5

9. Blurred or impaired vision and/or other visual disturbances 5

10. Numbness of the arm, hand, or shoulder preceding the headaches 5

11. Headaches, which last over two days 5

Your Score:_____

Scoring

5 to 15 points   *Mild Migraines.* If you scored in this category, you are fortunate. The migraines you experience are mild and infrequent. Thus, physical damage is unlikely, and with proper treatment they should be easily eradicated.

20 to 35 points *Moderate Migraine Illness:* At this level the migraines are usually severe enough to impair daily activity and to negatively affect lifestyle. If untreated, permanent damage to the brain may occur, including loss of peripheral vision, blood vessel weakness, and memory loss. Every effort should be made to eliminate the headaches before they worsen or before physical damage occurs.

40 to 55 points *Severe Migraine Illness:* The consequences of migraine attacks of this severity should be taken seriously. If untreated, permanent damage to the brain may occur, including loss of peripheral vision, blood vessel weakness, and memory loss. Every effort should be made to determine why they exist, then work towards a plan of reducing their frequency and severity. Usually, the frequency of the headaches can be significantly reduced. In many patients the headaches can be eliminated entirely.

60 and above *Extremely Severe Migraine Illness:* Warning: unless this condition is resolved, tissue damage of the brain membranes and eyes will occur. People in this category have migraines severe enough that tissue damage is inevitable. Most of these patients are taking high doses of medications, which aggravate the damage. The fact is the regular intake of strong painkillers directly damages the internal organs. Thus, it is important to immediately determine the cause of the migraines and institute aggressive treatment—without dangerous drugs.

If the reader scores positive for significant migraines, he/she must understand that a "paper diagnosis" is, by itself, insufficient. Laboratory tests must be performed for confirmation. These tests may include evaluation of glandular function, especially thyroid and adrenal function, plus food intolerance testing.

It is of utmost importance that the patient continues the search for the cause of his/her migraines. This is because only once the cause is determined can the cure be achieved. The practitioner of the healing arts must assist the patient in this effort. There is always a cause. If the physician or practitioner is unable to help, then the responsibility is up to the individual. The remaining chapters will help solve this riddle and put a halt to the endless searching.

Chapter 2

Many Kinds, Many Causes

There are many types of headaches. Doctors are taught early in their training to categorize them into one of three principal groups: tension headaches, migraine headaches, and cluster headaches. Other categories exist, but they are the more rare causes of headaches, representing 2% or less of the total headache occurrences. Included are headaches due to blood clots in the brain, traumatic headaches from severe injuries, such as concussions, brain infection headaches (meningitis/encephalitis), and the headaches of brain tumor. Headaches related to relatively common medical disorders represent a larger percentage. Diseases and/or illnesses known to produce headaches include high blood pressure, lung disease, hypothyroidism, Cushing's disease, hypoglycemia, and infections (fevers). Of note, over one half of patients with high blood pressure complain of headaches.

In the last 20 years a new category has been added to the list: premenstrual headache. This headache, which is common, occurs either just prior to or during menstruation.

Modern medicine excels in accurate diagnosis of the serious causes of headache. However, it often fails to discern the factors which generate the more common ones. Thus, the cause of tension, migraine, premenstrual, and cluster headaches remains elusive and the treatment poor. The majority of headache sufferers are left seemingly abandoned, wandering to and fro between the doctor, hospital, pharmacist, psychiatrist, acupuncturist, chiropractor, physical therapist, or masseuse. The approach of modern medicine to chronic headache is probably best exemplified by this quotation from *Harrison's Textbook of Internal Medicine:* "adolescents with daily frontal headaches . . . anxiety or tension is a probable factor. Equally puzzling is the somber, tense adult whose primary complaint is headache, or the migrainous person who in late life or at menopause begins to have daily headaches. *Here it becomes important to assess mental status . . . looking for evidences of anxiety, depression and hypochondriasis (italics mine)."* In contrast, it can be presumed that anyone with unexplainable chronic headaches or head pain would automatically and understandably become anxious and depressed—or even hypochondriacal—especially if that pain occurred on a daily basis. Thus, modern medicine has helped perpetuate the anxiety of such sufferers by claiming that this illness may be psychological. Yet, the fact is migraine is a physical rather than mental disease. Just as there are many kinds of headaches, there are many factors which cause them.

As stated previously there are common and rare causes. All must be considered in the evaluation of headache, although the history should serve as a guide for determining which approach to take. One need not always immediately rush the patient into the x-ray room and irradiate him/her with cranial x-rays, brain scans, and CAT scans at the first sign of a headache. On the other hand these tools may be invaluable to rule out serious underlying disease. The key is to use good sense, a concept known in medicine as *clinical judgment.* There is another factor. It is peace of mind. It may be necessary to rule out intracranial causes of headaches, including brain tumor, that is to reassure patients that no such lesion exists, even if the headache fits a "less serious" symptom pattern. Then again, anyone, even the most astute clinician, may err. There is no reason to take risks. However, the vast majority of headaches are due to causes other than brain tumors. Good judgment is one thing; paranoia is another.

There are a number of non-pathological causes of headaches. The most significant of these are listed as follows:

1. allergies to foods and chemicals

2. non-allergic chemical sensitivity

3. structural defects and/or muscle tension

4. hormonal disorders

5. blood sugar disturbances

6. digestive disturbances

7. infections (such as colds and flu)

8. stress

9. toxic exposure

10. sinus infections

Notice that psychological disorders, such as anxiety and depression, are not listed. This is because mental disorders per se are far from the major causes. Again, headaches are *physical* in nature, as will be demonstrated throughout this book.

Notice item Number 1: Allergy. There are literally hundreds, in fact, thousands, of allergic and chemical triggers. As will be discussed in greater detail in the following chapter, this appears to be the most common cause. In other words, migraines are largely caused by toxic reactions to what people breathe, drink, and eat. Migraineurs also suffer structural defects, hormonal disturbances, and digestive problems. Thus, migraine is more often the result of a combination of disorders rather than from any single cause. For instance, women with chronic migraines nearly always suffer from a combination of allergies plus hormonal problems. Regarding blood sugar and digestive disturbances, virtually all Americans have them.

Item Number 2, non-allergic chemical sensitivity, represents a significant cause. Categories of chemicals include those which are ingested via food and water, those which are inhaled, and those which are contacted and absorbed through the skin. Fumes are especially likely to trigger headaches, and this occurs for several reasons. Fumes gain direct access to the brain through the nose. At the roof of the nasal cavity there is a tiny thin bony membrane coated with paper-thin nerves. This is the cribiform plate. It is the brain's window to the outside world, and it is the sensory apparatus for smell. Volatile components readily penetrate it, entering the brain. Fumes are by nature volatile. Once inhaled, toxic components in the air may readily pass through the membrane and enter the brain. Headaches may result. There is another mechanism. If the fumes contain carbon monoxide, a highly toxic and potentially lethal gas, the headache can be devastating and prolonged, since this gas directly binds to red blood cells, poisoning them.

Most people are familiar with the cousin of carbon monoxide, that is *carbon dioxide*. The latter has the chemical formula, CO_2. The chemical formula for carbon monoxide is CO: it is missing an oxygen. This is what makes it so toxic. Upon entering the bloodstream, carbon monoxide seeks oxygen. Where is the most likely place to get it? It is the hemoglobin found in red blood cells, the natural carrier of oxygen. For every molecule of CO inhaled, one molecule of the red blood cell's hemoglobin is neutralized. In essence, carbon monoxide latches onto the hemoglobin molecule and ties up the oxygen, so that it cannot be used. This chemical vice grip is extremely difficult to break, and the chemical reaction between CO and the red cell is termed in medical textbooks as *irreversible*. The fact is this binding makes it impossible for the red cell to pick up oxygen when it passes through the lungs. One breath of contaminated air leads to the absorption of millions of carbon monoxide molecules. Within minutes most of the body's red cells can be poisoned. The result is oxygen depletion within the tissues, including the number one oxygen consumer, the brain. Fatigue, sleepiness, vague headache, and, in the case of prolonged and heavy exposure, death, may result. Here is the point. Headaches may be caused by toxic fumes from a leaky gas stove or water heater, a car-filled street, buses, airplane exhaust, or any other source which permeates the home or business. Formaldehyde gases, diesel fumes, car exhaust, sulfur dioxide, chlorine gas, and many other gaseous compounds are also known to provoke or aggravate headaches, because such chemicals also readily damage red cells.

There are hundreds and even thousands of chemicals which can cause headaches. What's more, untold thousands of chemicals, many of them outright toxins, are added to the food supply. This is tyranny, because people put their trust in the commercial food supply. If it is packaged as a "food," the majority of people would never believe it could be anything other than "safe." The role played by food additives in migraines will be described in detail in the next chapter. It is appropriate to list here the industrial, commercial, and agricultural chemicals which can generate toxic headaches:

Industrial/Commercial

- Kerosene
- Gasoline
- Benzene
- Dioxin
- Carbon tetrachloride
- Fluoride
- Industrial cleaners
- Bromine (or its gas)
- Formaldehyde (or its gas)
- Methyl chloride (or its gas)
- Chlorine (or its gas)
- Paints and paint fumes
- Solvents
- PCBs

Agricultural

- Nitrates and nitrites
- Pesticides
- Herbicides
- Fungicides
- Larvacides
- Fumigants

This list demonstrates how toxic the human environment is. Such toxins readily gain contact with the human cells, organs, and, particularly, the brain. This is evidence that headaches are largely a result of the environment. The number of headaches a person suffers may largely depend on how toxic that environment is. Toxicity in the workplace or even at home is a major cause of chronic headaches.

Heavy Metals

In industrialized countries heavy metal toxicity is a common cause of chronic illness. Since the turn of the century levels of aluminum, mercury, cadmium, arsenic, lead, and nickel have increased in the food and water by several hundred percent. Headaches are one of the most frequent symptoms of heavy metal toxicity. Lead, copper, arsenic, and mercury poisoning all commonly result in headaches.

Heavy metal poisoning should always be considered as a potential cause of chronic headaches, particularly in those headaches which elude diagnosis. This is especially true of headaches which are persistent, that is daily or weekly headaches. The fact is the daily dull type of headache which is persistent is a classical symptom of lead poisoning.

Heavy metals exert their toxic effects largely by poisoning the nerve cells. For instance, research indicates that copper can provoke a certain type of migraine by interfering with the transmission of nerve impulses in the brain. However, the same is true of mercury and lead, since both have a high affinity for nerve tissues and are, therefore, likely to disrupt the function of the brain and spinal nerves. Thus, the chronic headaches of heavy metal poisoning are primarily due to heavy metal overload of the brain. Once fixed within brain tissue these heavy metals greatly interfere with the transmission of impulses, causing a wide range of symptoms, including numbness, tingling, muscle weakness, muscle atrophy, loss of nerve or muscle control, and of course headaches.

Today, there is an epidemic which is out of control: mercury poisoning. The latest evidence implicates the contamination of fish, especially large ocean fish, as the culprit. Mercury is released into the environment from man-made pollution. It accumulates in the ocean. Here, bacteria absorb it, which are consumed by tiny ocean creatures. These creatures are then eaten by small fish, which are eaten by large fish. The mercury accumulates in the flesh and organs of the large fish, which humans consume. The result is nerve poisoning. Fish exceptionally high in mercury include swordfish, marlin, albacore tuna, bluefish, and king salmon. Other potentially toxic fish include yellow fin tuna, shark, and halibut.

Government research indicates that mercury levels in heavy fish eaters is several times higher than in moderate fish eaters. Hair analysis is an excellent screen for heavy metal exposure (see Chapter Three).

Drugs and Other Chemicals

It is true that a wide range of synthetic chemicals can provoke headaches, however, so can certain natural chemicals. Cigarette smoke, ergotamine, aflatoxin, biological amines (found in wines and cheeses), alkaloids (found in herbs and spices), and nitrates are examples of naturally occurring toxins capable of initiating headaches, particularly migraines—often within minutes of exposure. These, too, directly interfere with brain and nerve chemistry.

Certain drugs cause headaches. Most notable are birth control pills (BCPs). In North America tens of millions of women take these pills. The Pill is not only a potent cause of headaches, but it also aggravates existing migraine conditions. Thus, in any younger women suffering from persistent headaches the Pill must be considered as a cause. Other drugs known to cause headaches include cortisone, Indocin, aspirin, Cardiazem, acetaminophen, Coumadin, and Hydralazine. In addition, megadoses of vitamin A over a prolonged period can cause headaches. Note that two of the most common agents used to treat migraine, aspirin and acetaminophen, can actually cause it. This response can be due to an allergy to the drug. Thus, if a person is sensitive to aspirin or acetaminophen, taking it during a migraine will act to prolong the attack and may even worsen the pain.

Many drugs which lower blood pressure also cause headaches. This is due to a reduction in blood flow to the brain. Diuretics operate via this mechanism, although they also cause deficiencies of headache-fighting minerals such as potassium, calcium, selenium, and magnesium. What's more, diuretics can cause a kind of brain dehydration, which may also result in chronic headaches. Water is needed for proper brain function. It helps deliver nutrients to brain cells, while removing toxins. Thus, dehydration is a relatively common cause of headaches.

Cigarette smoke is a common cause of headaches. This is true both in smokers and in passive inhalers. One study performed in Britain showed that over 50% of smokers became headache-free, just by quitting. This indicates that smokers are allergic to the tobacco leaf and also to the smoke that is generated from it. For birth control pill users similar results are seen, with over 30% being relieved of their headaches after discontinuing the pill.

The Role of Stress

Many people assume that headaches are the result of stress. Others know of no obvious stressor that provokes them, rather, believing that the stress they experience is due to headaches. The fact is there is some truth in both these concepts. Certainly, stress can provoke headaches. Yet, it is the premise of this book that, contrary to popular belief, stress is far from the primary cause. Other factors, particularly food allergy, chemical sensitivity, hormonal imbalances, toxic metal overload, and nutritional deficiencies, are far more significant.

One important question is, how can stress cause headaches? Mental stress initiates a wide array of physical responses. Both physical and mental stress weaken a person's defenses. Whenever an individual is stressed, strain is placed upon internal organs such as the immune system, digestive tract, liver, pancreas, thyroid, and adrenals. This is mediated via the central nervous system, i.e. the CNS, the region first affected by stress. The CNS sends nerve impulses in response to our thoughts to the various organs and glands. Positive thoughts result in the delivery of useful impulses, and negative thoughts deliver harmful ones. If the negative or stressful thoughts are severe and prolonged, symptoms and even disease may result. What's more, stress greatly affects the muscles and nerves, causing tightening of the muscles, especially those of the back, neck, and scalp. This is usually how stress leads to headaches.

The ill effects of stress differ from person to person. Everyone is subjected to it, every day. Our thoughts can either neutralize or aggravate these unavoidable stresses. It is important to minimize the ill effects of stress. In order to do so, it is helpful to study some of the natural anti-stress mechanisms.

When the mind entertains a stressful thought, numerous physiological reactions begin to occur. Impulses arising in the brain are delivered directly to the internal organs through the spinal cord and peripheral nerves. The stomach responds with the secretion of hydrochloric acid. The liver responds by synthesizing sugar, or, in the case in chronic stress, by increasing the synthesis of cholesterol. The adrenal glands react by increasing the production of adrenaline and other adrenal hormones, such as cortisone. The pancreas secretes more insulin, and the thyroid increases the output of thyroid hormone. The thymus, that all-important immune gland located behind the sternum, shrinks. The circulatory system reacts with a constriction of blood vessels, leading to a reduction of oxygen to the tissues, including the brain. The lack of oxygen aggravates the brain tissue, resulting in headaches, dizziness, and sluggish mental function. The nerves become agitated, sending strong messages to the muscles. When the muscles tighten, the nerves are impinged, causing pain. Here's how this happens. When the brain receives stressful messages due to mental pressures, it sends impulses down the spinal cord. These messages are carried through nerves leaving the cord to the muscles. These stress-induced messages cause the muscles to tighten, leading to torque. Both joint and muscle damage may result, plus the torque reduces blood flow. It is the pressure, that is torque, on the nerves, along with the reduction in blood flow, which causes the pain. This is descriptively known as *tension headache*.

Stress, Blood Sugar, and Migraine

The blood sugar mechanism is intricately involved in brain function. This is because the organ relies primarily upon sugar as its fuel. Stress greatly disrupts blood sugar, leading to either a sudden decline or in the extreme a sudden rise, as in diabetes.

The brain is greatly affected by any disruption in blood sugar, since all its cells depend upon glucose, which is the normal fuel in the blood. A sudden drop in blood sugar levels negatively affects the brain. Often, the result is a variety of symptoms, which may include depression, anxiety, severe pain, and migraines. Regarding migraines it is the sudden drop in blood sugar which is of concern. Stress readily causes such sudden drops.

There is another critical factor. This relates to the adrenal glands, which are extensively involved in controlling blood sugar. The adrenal glands are greatly damaged by stress. Whether the adrenal abuse is due to physical or mental stress, the result is the same: an increase in the secretion of adrenal hormones, resulting in either a sudden drop in blood sugar levels or the inability to maintain adequate levels. Eventually, as a consequence of stress-induced depletion of the hormones the adrenal glands are no longer able to produce adequate amounts of hormones. This subject will be discussed in greater detail in Chapter Five.

Both the pancreas and the liver help manage blood sugar levels. The pancreas is especially important, since it produces insulin. This is the primary hormone for regulating blood sugar levels. Stress often leads to the production of excess amounts of insulin. The combination of the stress-induced secretion of adrenal hormones and insulin into the bloodstream can spell serious trouble for the brain. This is because an excess of these hormones causes blood sugar levels to drop suddenly. When the brain is deprived of glucose, which is its primary fuel, headaches often result.

Yet, stress merely precipitates the headaches. Thus, if the underlying problems are corrected, the headaches are resolved, *even if the stress remains the same.* Even so, it is advised that all highly stressed individuals learn new ways to cope with their problems. Stress is highly destructive. It always leads to physiological damage. It serves no useful function. The fact is, frequently, it even kills.

Intestinal Reflexes

Irritants in the stomach or intestines cause headaches. There is a unique relationship between the head and gut, which is maintained by the vagus nerve.

The vagus is classified as a cranial nerve. This means that it arises within the brain. The nerve exits directly from the skull, without going into the spinal cord. It is the main nerve supply to the stomach, intestines, liver, pancreas, and colon. As it descends it divides into several branches, including some in the neck.

The vagus is a powerful nerve. When it becomes irritated, it can produce a variety of symptoms. One of them is head pain. How does this occur? The vagus is not a pain nerve per se. When it is irritated, what does result is a form of referred pain, known medically as *vagal cephalgia*. This term defines scalp pain and/or headaches of vagal origin. Thus, in many cases headaches may be caused by disordered digestion. If the cause of the vagus nerve irritation is eliminated, the pain will recede. For instance, if the stomach is inflamed, nerve fibers arising from it may refer pain to the scalp, particularly the scalp on top of the head. If the inflammation is treated with agents specific for stomach disorders, such as ginger or licorice root, the head pain often disappears. Or, if the stomach is infected, for instance, by *Helicobacter pylori*—the cause of stomach ulcers—this may cause inflammation, leading to headaches. If the infection is eliminated, for instance with oil of wild oregano, then as a result, headaches disappear. A more dramatic example occurs within the colon. It too contains vagal nerve fibers, which, when irritated, produce referred pain. In this case pain may be on the top of the head and also quite often in the rear or occipital region. This is known as colonic cephalgia.

The most common cause of *colonic cephalgia* is constipation. A plugged up bowel can cause headaches simply by increasing mechanical pressure on colonic nerves. When the pressure is released, as occurs with a healthy bowel movement, the headache or head pain dramatically disappears. Some believe that constipation causes headaches primarily by intoxication, that is, the pollution of the blood by one's own wastes. While this can occur, such headaches are more commonly due to mechanical factors. This was proven by Dr. Alvarez of the Mayo Clinic. He reproduced headaches in susceptible patients by stuffing cotton in their rectums. Thus, certainly, constipation is a major cause of headaches. What's more, its role is easily proven. This is because as soon as the mechanical issue is resolved, the headaches disappear. Thus, in the headache prevention plan proper normal elimination is essential.

A great deal can be done to prevent constipation-induced headaches. Here are some useful measures:

1. Answer the call of nature whenever it occurs. Avoid "holding it." Go when you need to go. This is a critical factor.

2. Go for a walk every day. The best anti-constipation exercise is a brisk walk in the morning before or after breakfast. The walk should be a minimum of 1/2 mile, although 1 to 2 miles is preferable. A daily two mile walk combined with the proper diet is a virtual guarantee for preventing constipation. Abdominal exercises are also effective.

3. Drink 6 large glasses of water daily (non-chlorinated) and eat water-retaining foods. Such foods retain moisture in the colon, and this creates stools which are bulky and soft. A partial list of these foods includes:

   • watermelon   • carrots
   • cantaloupe   • lettuce
   • honeydew melon   • celery

- citrus fruits
- kiwi
- grapes
- apples
- pears
- tomatoes
- cucumbers
- eggplant
- cabbage
- endive
- parsley
- pea pods
- water chestnuts
- turnips
- watercress
- onions
- spinach
- squash
- radishes

4. Take supplemental fiber sources. The extra fiber should be consumed daily. Good sources of fiber include:

- bran, especially oat, corn, barley, and rice
- psyllium husk and seed
- alfalfa
- fruit pectin
- vegetable fibers

Note: many people are allergic to grains and, thus, the brans of such grains would be contraindicated. In fact, in some individuals by eating such grains the constipation is aggravated. The most well-tolerated is rice bran. In virtually all instances wheat bran should be strictly avoided. Incredibly, the latter is a major cause of constipation.

5. Take an acidophilus supplement with potent implanting capacity, such as Health-Bac, which is based upon extensive European research. Up to 90% of the bulk of the normal stool consists of bacteria. Thus, Health-Bac can be used to naturally improve the flow of stools. This is because the natural bacteria, which grow within the intestines profusely, will add to the bulk of the stool and assist in easing elimination.

6. Take a liver/bile purifying supplement. This is because the bile and liver secretions are critical to proper digestion as well as stool formation. The Cell-u-Clenz wild greens drops are an excellent type of liver/bile-activating agent. Made from wild-grown greens found in remote regions it has a potent, dependable action in the liver and gallbladder. For optimal results take two or more droppersful daily. It may also be used in a gallbladder purge. Simply add four to six droppersful of the Powerdrops to 1/4 cup extra virgin olive oil plus 1/4 cup high quality apple cider or balsamic vinegar. For an anti-constipation liver cleanse drink 1/4 to 1/2 cup of this mixture daily. This formula will aggressively purge toxins from the liver, resulting in normalization of function as well as an improvement in overall health. The wild greens are a powerful natural medicine, one of the most rare and valuable ever produced. Since its ingredients are exclusively hand picked from the wild it is highly rare: only a few thousand bottles are produced every year. This is the most effective anti-constipation therapy available. The wild green drops are available mainly by mail-order: 1-800-243-5242. The drops themselves, when taken sublingually, are effective for headache relief.

It is critical to become educated about all the various types of headaches. However, it is difficult for the headache patient to pin down precisely what might be causing his/her symptoms/disease, that is without medical help. This issue will be addressed in the following chapter.

Chapter 3

Making the Diagnosis

Headache sufferers face a major dilemma. They know their pain is real. To be rid of it is their goal, one which they pursue with great effort. Usually, they have no clue regarding what brings on the headaches. To complicate matters the medical profession has difficulty finding any answers, unless a diagnosis of organic disease can be made. As a rule medical doctors or, for that matter, other health professionals, such as chiropractors, osteopathic physicians, acupuncturists, and dentists, really have no idea what to do. They may wish to help the patient but often find that they have few directions in which to turn. This chapter has been designed for these doctors and for concerned patients. The scientific evidence dictates that migraines have a biological cause. It is likely that many health practitioners will agree with this and wish to learn all they can about innovative methods for treating this pervasive illness.

An engineer must first determine the source of a bridge's weakness before he can rebuild it. A TV repairman must find out why a unit is defective before it can be fixed. An auto mechanic must make a diagnosis concerning a defective engine before he can begin repairs. The same should hold true in the medical field. Such was the philosophy of Andrew Taylor Still,

M.D., the founder of Osteopathic Medicine, who said in relation to human illness, "Find it, fix it, and leave it alone."

Modern or Western medicine is one of the few medical systems which treats symptoms instead of causes. Both East Indian and Chinese medicine attempt to search for the cause. The ancient Greeks made a partial attempt to determine causes, although their system was greatly improved during the Middle Ages by Islamic doctors, who were thorough cause-seekers. While the Greeks were largely arm-chair physicians according to K. Khaleel, in his book, *Science in the Name of God,* it was Islamic physicians who invented the scientific method in medicine. American Indian medicine is cause-oriented, as are many of the medicinal approaches of South American societies such as the Incas.

The American Indians, the original inhabitants of North and South America, were a people largely in tune with nature. In the realm of the healing arts they utilized naturally occurring substances—foods, food extracts, and herbs. Often, they administered highly specific therapies in their attempts to cure illness. Many of these remedies are only now being recognized for their curative potential.

If this has been man's historical tendency, why is there such a deficiency of this philosophy in the current forms of medicine? If anything, we should be further advanced in using the scientific method to determine cause and effect. Considering the advancements of modern science the determination of what is causing a given person's headaches, and, thus, the accomplishment of its final cure should be a rapid, efficient, and effective process. This should be the status quo. Instead, the patient with migraine is often confronted with a barrage of futile questions and/or undergoes a battery of inconclusive tests. Usually, the medical effort amounts to little more than a random attempt to reassure the concerned patient that, "Nothing serious is wrong." Once all the obvious medical causes are ruled out, the frustrated physician may proclaim, "It's all in your head" or "You're under too much stress." As a result, the patient is often referred to a psychiatrist. Some people are even blamed for their headaches—as if they created them on purpose. The scenario is something like this, "You are holding onto your pain for some emotional reason." This is mere nonsense. It is important to avoid taking these comments personally, as the doctor is probably so frustrated that he/she just doesn't know what else to do. The tipoff to this medical frustration is the question, "Are you having personal problems?" You can imagine what the next suggestion will be.

Yet, recently positive changes have occurred. For instance, numerous physicians are familiar with the role of food allergy in migraine. Thus, it is common for doctors to take at least a minimal dietary history, recommending against the typical provocative foods or other substances: cheese, chocolate, red wine, MSG, etc.

The physician must be aggressive at determining the underlying cause of a migraine. He/she should perform a thorough history and physical examination and run the appropriate tests. CAT scans, MRIs, and other highly invasive or potentially toxic scans are rarely needed; they are usually over-prescribed. Here, as in many diseases the most important method is neglected: a careful history.

During their training medical students are taught that the history is the most important part of any evaluation. While this is true of many diseases, there is a special variation which applies to patients with chronic migraines. As a rule, the most important step in diagnosing and curing migraines is laboratory testing. This means that tests are more revealing in achieving a migraine cure than are the history and physical. However, it must be noted that a thorough history and complete physical exam are mandatory in any migraine evaluation. Great care must be taken to insure that the headaches are not due to serious or life-threatening disease, and a thorough history and physical are the best ways to do this.

Through these three methods—the history, the physical and the tests—the sufferer can usually determine whether his/her worst fears are true. Is there any hope? Are the headaches simply a result of stress, or is there an underlying cause? Are the migraines a consequence of serious and life-threatening disease, or is the problem a simple and curable one? Are the headaches a result of psychological disturbances, or are they simply the manifestation of a malingering hypochondriac? Many migraine patients have been so labeled.

How to Make a Diagnosis

Headaches can be a symptom of serious, underlying disease. Most people are aware of the life-threatening causes of headaches such as brain tumors, cancer, stroke, aneurysm, cerebral hemorrhage, and meningitis. Many of these conditions are associated with a sudden onset of symptoms, although a few, such as certain brain tumors, can exhibit symptoms over a prolonged period. These symptoms of an undiagnosed brain tumor might include severe pain, headache, nausea, vomiting, dizziness, loss of consciousness, extremely stiff neck, and visual loss. Such symptoms, especially if acute or following injury, require medical diagnosis and treatment. It is possible that certain people will become overly concerned by this statement, since some of the aforementioned symptoms occur in migraines of non-serious origin. However, fortunately, most migraine sufferers have long-since had these serious conditions ruled out. For that majority other less ominous disorders are responsible.

Types of Tests

There are six major categories of tests useful for evaluating migraines. These categories are as follows:

1. *Tests to rule out serious causes.* These include CAT scans, MRIs, brain scans, X-rays, EEGs, angiographs, and certain blood tests.

2. *Food allergy testing.* The recommended test involves highly sophisticated, specialized blood testing for immune allergy reactions to numerous foods (for more details on a highly accurate method of food allergy testing see page 51).

3. *Vitamin/mineral assessment.* This is done primarily through blood, hair, and urine analysis.

4. *Digestive analysis.* This is done via blood, urine, and stool assays.

5. *Hormonal gland function.* This is accomplished through high-tech blood and urine analysis, as well as highly accurate historical or symptom tests, that is questionnaires.

6. *Toxic Metal Analysis.* This is done primarily through analyzing hair or tissue samples, although symptom analysis, blood and urine samples are occasionally used.

These tests can be utilized to diagnose the majority of migraines. For most patients tests in the first category will be negative. Nearly all will have significant allergies, and many will test positive for nutritional deficiencies, digestive disturbances, and hormonal dysfunction.

One of the last stages in establishing the diagnosis is selecting the medical terminology. Everyone is interested in knowing his/her diagnosis. According to the system promulgated in this book the chronic migraine sufferer will rarely qualify for only one diagnosis. The typical case is similar to this: MIGRAINE HEADACHE, HYPOTHYROIDISM, FOOD ALLERGIES, and INTESTINAL MALABSORPTION. Other diagnoses commonly determined in migraine patients include adrenal cortical insufficiency, intestinal parasites, anemia, thyroiditis, hypertension, carbohydrate intolerance, lead poisoning, mercury poisoning, cadmium poisoning, *Candida albicans*, and hypertension (i.e. high blood pressure).

For any health practitioner as well as patient, the basic goal should be the elimination of the headaches. In the majority of cases this is possible. In a few instances the best that can be accomplished is to reduce their severity and frequency, so that life can become more tolerable. Thus, both the patient and the physician must be persistent in the objective to discover the cause, as well as the cure, of this disease.

There are millions of people whose lives are disabled by migraine headache pain. Headaches draw the fun out of life. They drain vitality and impair productivity. Just as the blood flow stagnates in the victims' brains, so do their lives. Every day for the individual mired in pain is a potentially useful day lost. The headache sufferer knows this all too well.

Making a diagnosis is not difficult. All the tools are available. Any physician can do it. Unfortunately, patients are at the mercy of a medical profession inadequately informed about the causation of disease. Finding a physician who is willing to pursue these angles or who has the expertise to do so is often a difficult task. A small list of physicians, medical institutions, and chiropractors capable of assisting the migraineur is provided in Appendix D. Chiropractors, while unable to perform many of the more sophisticated medical tests, are allowed to draw blood in certain states and are skilled in some of the structural therapies described in this book. The ideal, of course, is to find a D.O. or an M.D. skilled in these techniques.

The pain and agony of migraines can be halted. Making the diagnosis helps stop this ongoing crisis by:

1. Giving the patient some firm answers, including medical diagnoses illustrating the cause.

2. Providing patients with effective cures.

3. Helping migraineurs to be more accurate observers. The more they know about what triggers their headaches, the easier it is to avoid them.

4. Giving both the physician and patient direction, so that a cure can be efficiently accomplished.

There is another critical element to consider: hope. For all diseases there is hope, that is if the correct diagnosis can be made and the proper therapy prescribed. The body has been constructed magnificently. It has inherent healing capacities. If these capacities can be strategically assisted, virtually any condition can be reversed, including migraine. The fact is migraines and other headaches are curable. Again, the key is to determine the exact cause and, thus, prescribe the precise therapy. However, the individual must maintain a positive attitude and believe in the possibilities. Think positive, have hope: soon, you will find the cure.

Chapter 4

Allergies:
The Number One Cause

In uncovering the mystery of migraines, allergies are the missing link. A person can be allergic to a wide range of toxins, inhalants, chemicals, and fumes. Incredibly, a greater number of migraines are caused by allergies to naturally occurring substances than by all those caused by synthetics, chemicals, drugs, and fumes combined. The fact is food allergies are the main culprit. People react to a wide range of foods. Allergies to natural beverages, such as coffee, cola, or tea, are also relatively common. Yet, could food, the nourishment for human survival, cause headaches? How can something natural and wholesome cause misery and pain? The mechanisms behind this are now well understood. Modern researchers have found that foods are made up of a complexity of compounds, many of which can cause the reactions, leading to inflammation as well as headaches.

The concept that food allergy is the major cause of migraines is far from a new discovery. Rather, as early as 1907 it was known that food allergies cause migraines. In 1936 Goltman wrote a monumental paper entitled, "Mechanism of

Migraine." In it he reported a case of a patient who was mistakenly subjected to brain surgery during a migraine crisis. The operation was performed during the migraine attack, and the surgeons were able to directly view what occurred. It was observed that the patient's brain and brain membranes were markedly swollen and inflamed, but no serious abnormality or disease was found.

Several days later it was determined that the patient was allergic to wheat. Amazingly, when the patient was challenged with wheat, similar swelling was palpable. This was easy to determine, since the surgery left a temporary opening in the skull.

The link between migraines and food allergies was largely neglected until the 1950s, when Leon Unger and Joel Cristol, both M.D.s, wrote their landmark article, "Allergic Migraine." This article appeared in the prominent medical journal, *Annals of Allergy*. The gist of the article is best described by these authors' own words: "Migraine is an allergic disease due to one or more foods." This is a profound statement. It is a statement that the medical profession is largely unaware of. Yet, the evidence is rather conclusive: there is a plethora of recent data offering the same conclusions. Migraine patients have suffered extensively and for too long. The irony is the evidence has been available all along. For instance, in an article published in 1921 in the *Journal of the American Medical Association* Dr. Brown claimed that diet played a role in migraines. In 1930 Dr. LaRoche and colleagues noted that foods cause migraines.

Numerous articles have been recently published in major medical journals describing the allergic link to migraines. The fact is hundreds of articles have proven an undeniable fact: that migraines are caused by food allergies until proven otherwise.

The Migraine Personality: Does it Really Exist?

The majority of psychologists and psychiatrists, as well as the majority of physicians, believe in what is called the *migraine personality*. This stereotype is thought to occur commonly in women, especially menstruating women, but it also may be ascribed to men. The women are supposedly perfectionists, who are obsessed with keeping everything in order to the tiniest detail at work or home. According to this theory the perfectionism causes emotional stress, which provokes migraines. Another female stereotype is the hypochondriac. A hypochondriac is defined as a person who complains of an illness which does not exist. Supposedly, migraineurs use their illness to accomplish everything from seeking attention to expressing anger over a forlorn relationship. In my experience nothing could be further from the truth. In fact, I have yet to see a single case of the migraine personality. My experience is far from isolated. It was Unger who previously fully confirmed this. "Although emotions can precipitate attacks, it *is only in those who are allergic to one or more foods*" [italics mine]. It was expected that Dr. Unger make this observation, since over 90% of his migraine patients showed either significant improvement or complete eradication of their headaches once the allergic foods were omitted from their diets. Some of the most formidable research on the food allergy migraine connection was done by Dr. Unger in 1952, when he determined that there are three types of migraines: 1) Those caused exclusively by foods 2) Those in which foods appear to play a minor role 3) Those caused by foods under certain conditions, including stress or exhaustion. Dr. Unger also discovered that certain chemicals, including chemical-based food additives, cause migraines. Some of the more common chemical agents that he determined as culprits include the following:

- alcohol
- nitrates (and nitrites)
- caffeine
- phenylethylamine
- tyramine
- monosodium glutamate (MSG)
- theobromine
- benzoic acid
- food dyes
- salicylates

Many of the above are common food additives which are extensively disguised in hundreds of foods. All aggressively provoke migraines. This demonstrates an ominous fact: migraine is largely a modern disease due to exposure to toxic chemicals. Freely added to food, such chemicals poison the digestive tract, internal organs, and nervous system, leading to headaches. These chemicals also readily poison the adrenal glands—also a major risk factor. Today, incredibly, there are over 6000 synthetic chemicals approved for addition to foods. The majority are known carcinogens. People suffer enormously from the burden of ingested toxins. What an injustice it is to put such chemicals in the foods, that is to purposely harm people with known poisons. The result is not only dire symptoms, such as headaches, but also outright disease, even sudden death. Diseases due to the ingestion of synthetic chemicals include:

- asthma
- attention deficit disorder
- autism
- arthritis
- bronchitis
- epilepsy
- cancer
- nephritis
- colitis
- gallbladder disorders
- Crohn's disease
- heart disorders
- hepatitis
- depression
- migraine
- seizures

The Allergy-Migraine Connection: A Review of Scientific Literature

Since the early 1950s numerous articles have been written concerning the connection between food, food additives and chemicals with migraines. Here are some of the key findings discussed in these articles:

1. In a study involving 43 adult migraine sufferers, Mansfield and associates reduced headache frequency by two thirds by removing suspected allergenic foods from the diet.

2. Dr. Vaughan found that nearly one half of patients with chronic migraine were aided, in terms of a reduction in the frequency and severity of headaches, when potentially allergenic foods, such as eggs, milk, corn, and wheat, were eliminated from the diet.

3. As early as 1921 researchers found chemicals in the blood of migraine patients which constricted arteries within the brain, leading to pain. Later it was found that these substances, serotonin and histamine, are the very chemicals which are liberated during allergic reactions.

4. Recently, it was discovered that migraine sufferers' platelets are more sticky than normal. These platelets clog circulation and may also release serotonin and other chemicals which are associated with the genesis of headache pain. It has long been known that allergic reactions cause platelets to become activated and "clump" together. This clumping blocks blood flow to the brain, leading to poor oxygen supply and, therefore, headaches.

5. Dr. Mansfield found that certain foods commonly cause migraines. These foods include milk, wheat, corn, eggs, soybeans, peanuts, chocolate, and alcoholic beverages. He

determined that eliminating these foods led to an improvement in the majority of cases.

6. In 1989 researchers at the Montefiore Medical Headache Unit in New York found that out of a total of 171 patients, approximately 50% reported alcohol as a precipitating factor for migraines. Nearly 10% identified NutraSweet as a trigger.

7. Dr. Ellen Grant of the Department of Neurology, Charing Cross Hospital, London, England, achieved a significant reduction in migraines via allergy removal. Of the 60 patients tested 50 became headache free, an 85% improvement. What's more, an unexpected benefit was seen. Of the 15 patients who had high blood pressure, all had normal blood pressure by the end of the study.

8. Concerning a concept first described by Rowe in 1931 it has been found that many people have allergies without realizing it and without obvious symptoms. The only way that an individual can experience a reaction to a hidden allergy is to eliminate the food from the diet for several weeks and then reintroduce it. Only then can obvious symptoms due to the food be produced. Chronic illnesses, including migraines, were found to be caused by these hidden food allergies.

9. Dr. Monro and colleagues found that two-thirds of severe migraine sufferers had food allergies and that these allergies were the primary cause of their headaches. This allergy-migraine connection was determined by a combination of allergy testing and food avoidance. The results of this study were reported in 1980 in the prominent British medical journal, *The Lancet*.

10. For years researchers have known that the risks of internal bleeding within the brain are greatly increased in users of birth control pills. Women who use the Pill are six times more likely to develop cerebral bleeding, and, if they also smoke, they are 22 times more likely. Based upon the Pill's adverse effects upon cerebral circulation, Dr. Ellen Grant felt an investigation of its effects upon migraine was warranted. The results were as would be expected. Women on the Pill had three times as many migraines as non-users. What's more, it was determined that these Pill-induced migraines can be both severe and damaging. Dr. Grant recorded the existence of actual tissue damage to arteries and veins within the brain. She also found that small arteries, known as arterioles, found within the pain-sensitive uterus were thicker in BCP users than non-users. Another abnormality was that the uterine veins were swollen and congested.

It would appear that evidence is accumulating that birth control pills are far more toxic than users realize. Dr. Grant feels that this toxicity is largely due to a bizarre alteration in liver function. In fact, if taken for prolonged periods, birth control pills can cause permanent liver damage.

11. In 1983 Dr. J. Egger and fellow researchers presented findings on the cause of childhood migraine which were published in a prominent British medical journal. This research was performed at the Hospital for Sick Children and Institute of Child Health in London, England. Their findings are summarized as follows: when allergenic foods were identified and removed, 93% of children with severe migraines recovered completely with no further headaches. What's more, other complaints and illnesses including asthma, behavioral disorders, stomach pain, and eczema were also improved or were eliminated.

By summarizing these findings a point has been made. These are legitimate, scientific studies performed by experienced researchers. In addition, all these studies were published in prominent medical journals. The evidence is clear: migraine headaches and food allergies are directly connected.

I have successfully treated over 400 cases of chronic migraine, which only further solidifies the truth of what these researchers have determined. Many of these patients have searched extensively for a cure. Nearly half experienced migraines for greater than 15 years. The majority have been to numerous doctors and medical clinics, spending uncountable thousands of dollars. Yet, all were either cured or considerably improved. The researchers quoted previously had similar dramatic results. Physicians should take note of a basic fact: patients who have migraines seek to be rid of their problem. For the physician to serve a useful function in regard to migraine patients, he/she must become familiarized with the role food allergies play in causing migraines.

The author of this book cannot possibly see all the migraine patients who exist. Therefore, the objective here is to provide both the lay person and the professional with convincing data that alternative therapies for migraines exist and that they are highly effective. The public desperately needs more open-minded, nutritionally oriented practitioners. It is difficult to find such physicians in a major metropolitan area, let alone rural regions or medium-sized cities. However, the awareness of the value of preventive and nutritional medicine is increasing.

Almost any food or beverage can cause migraines. To many this may seem overwhelming. It could be, if you were to attempt to determine the allergies on your own. This is a difficult, time-consuming, and inaccurate method for diagnosing food allergies. The easiest way to isolate allergenic foods is to utilize diagnostic allergy testing. Ideally, it is necessary to find a physician who specializes in natural medicine and who is open to the treatment described in this book. Plus, regarding allergy testing the most effective test—the one I used to successfully treat my patients—is only performed by one lab. Any doctor can order it, even your family doctor, who is possibly unfamiliar with this method. It merely requires a tube of blood using a specialized preservative. For more information regarding this test call 1-800-243-5242.

Many migraineurs who believe they have allergies think they know what their allergies are. This is highly unlikely. Why would anyone want to rack his/her brain trying to figure out the allergenic foods, especially when the technology exists to find out precisely what these food allergies are? This point is stressed, because many patients resist the idea that they might have hidden food allergies that could cause migraines. When confronted with the prospect that allergies could be involved, they often proclaim, "I already know what my allergies are." Or, "I don't have allergies." Both claims are erroneous in terms of science and in respect to migraine tendencies. One can be entirely free of common allergy symptoms, such as runny nose, hives, itching, and rash, but still have numerous allergies. I have yet to meet a migraine sufferer who truly knew even a few of his/her allergies, let alone comprehend them all. With the huge variety of food and food additives which are consumed, it is difficult to make such a determination. There are a few exceptionally perceptive individuals who have linked an occasional headache to its cause. Yet, even with these rare people, the origins of the majority of their headaches still elude them.

The Food Intolerance Test—A Simple Method for Determining Migraine-Provoking Foods

Many migraine patients have undergone allergy testing. However, even after removing the suspect foods they still have migraines. This makes sense. There are hundreds of common foods and food additives. How can anyone determine for certain which they are allergic to? Others have never had an allergy test. In either case the Food Intolerance Test can prove to be invaluable.

By determining the causative allergies, this test has saved innumerable migraine patients from continual pain and suffering. It is best described as a specialized blood test for diagnosing food, chemical, and beverage allergies, and is perhaps the easiest of all allergy tests to perform. All that is required is the drawing of a single tube of blood done as a fasting sample. What supersedes its simplicity is its accuracy, which is nearly 80%. By comparison, scratch testing is 20% to 40% accurate, while RAST testing (for foods) is only about 5% to 15% accurate. The ELISA test, a complex blood test which is relatively new, has been highly touted. However, its accuracy is less than 40%, and only a comparatively few foods are included in the evaluation.

There is yet another allergy testing method. This is fasting followed by a rotation diet. This method was originally pioneered by the respected allergist, Theron Randolph, M.D. The idea is to go on a complete fast for 3 to 5 days to clear out all reactive compounds from the body. Then, on an empty stomach suspect foods are introduced, one at a time. The patient awaits a measurable reaction such as runny nose, rash, irritability, headache, diarrhea, fatigue, etc. If such symptoms occur, the food is deemed responsible. This is an honorable method. However, it has its limitations. Incredibly, through this method it would take nearly a year to investigate the hundreds of foods and food additives commonly found in the diet. The cycle of fasting and adding back of foods would have to be repeated over and over again. In addition, delayed reactions of up to three to four days after food consumption make it difficult to pinpoint the offending food/beverage. In other words, even a fasting challenge with a specific food may not produce obvious symptoms, even though the food is potentially toxic.

The Food Intolerance Test solves these dilemmas. Overall, its advantages are as follows:

1) It is simple to perform

2) It is accurate

3) It has a proven track record—thousands of migraine patients have benefited

4) It is cost-effective

In terms of price the Food Intolerance Test is truly a value for the money. The cost is approximately $2.00 per food. By comparison, RAST testing costs $8.00 to $12.00 per food, and ELISA costs a minimum of $6.00. Scratch testing may be even more costly.

How the Test is Performed

The test is performed by drawing blood in a special tube which contains a unique preservative. This preservative keeps the human blood cells alive during storage and transport. Once received, the blood is mixed with food extracts. Through a special high powered microscope the technician views the interactions and physiological changes that occur within the blood as a result of the food antigen-immune reactions and records them according to severity. Reactions are graded 1, 2 or 3, with the latter being most severe.

A variety of observations are made depending upon the intensity of the immunological reactions. A list of the possibilities includes:

1) inflammation

2) clumping of red blood cells

3) clumping of platelets

4) damage to cell membranes

5) reduction in white blood cell mobility

6) destruction of white blood cells

Severe allergic reactions can be associated with inflammation, cell damage, and even cell death. The same processes also occur in the living state. Remember, this test is done on *live cells*, freshly taken from the human body. It takes little imagination to understand why such allergic reactions produce migraines. Experience with patients proves that mild, moderate, and severe reactions all can cause headaches. Sometimes, a person can eat a food to which he/she is mildly allergic without having a headache. However, on other occasions migraine is provoked. This may depend upon how stressed an individual's system might be on any given day. A person's stress can vary by the hour, by the minute, or even by the second. Severe stress greatly increases the vulnerability to toxic reactions.

How Food Allergy Reactions Occur: The Immune Connection

Once it was thought that nearly all allergies were the result of immune reactions against proteins. These proteins are known immunologically as *antigens*. While it is true that protein or antigen-immune reactions account for many allergic responses, it is now known that a variety of allergic reactions can occur as a result of ingesting foods or chemicals devoid of protein. Examples of non-protein substances which can evoke allergic reactions include alcohol, sugar, corn syrup, sulfites, alkaloids, NutraSweet, and saccharin.

It must be stressed that the protein-antigen reaction mechanism remains a common and extremely important cause of allergic illness. Let's examine how this reaction occurs.

High protein foods are complex compounds made up of untold numbers of protein molecules bound together by molecular bonds. Consider a fish fillet, for example. Its useful nutritional components must be liberated by digestive juices in the stomach and intestines. The pancreas secretes potent enzymes, which along with the hydrochloric acid of the stomach act to break proteins into simpler compounds. Proper function of this digestive process is critical in order to remain healthy. The tendency to develop allergic reactions to protein is directly related to how thoroughly it is digested. Sluggish or impaired digestion leads to the incomplete breakdown of food. This results in abnormal protein compounds, which elicits allergic reactions. The abnormal proteins, once absorbed into the bloodstream, greatly aggravate the immune system, causing the toxic reactions typical of food allergies.

It was once thought that protein could be absorbed only if it was completely digested into its component parts known as amino acids. This theory held that only amino acids could be transported from the intestines into the bloodstream. Larger molecules were supposedly prohibited from entry. Now it is known that this theory is wrong. Hundreds of scientific papers have demonstrated that incompletely digested protein molecules, literally undigested food, can be absorbed into the blood and that such proteins greatly increase the vulnerability to food intolerance and immune attack. In migraine this is precisely what occurs; the inappropriately digested protein is regarded as a foreign substance and is attacked by the immune defenses.

White blood cells surround these proteins in order to digest and detoxify them. The immune system also reacts by producing special anti-allergy proteins known as immunoglobulins. Several types of immunoglobulins exist. They are known by the abbreviations IgG, IgM, IgD, IgE, and IgA. Of these the most important, in terms of allergic defenses, are IgE, IgG, and IgA.

In respect to chronic food allergy IgG and IgA are most important. They are produced by special white blood cells known as B-lymphocytes. These lymphocytes are located throughout the body, but heavy concentrations are found within the intestinal walls, in lymph nodes, and within the spleen and liver. As such, the B-lymphocytes are strategically located for intercepting bacteria, viruses, yeasts, parasites, or allergens—anything which might illicit an immune response. Plus, the B-cells are immunospecific. This means that they will produce a different immunoglobulin for each immune stimulus. Thus, there are anti-bacterial, anti-viral, anti-yeast, anti-parasitic, and, yes, anti-food, immunoglobulins. In the utterly astounding complexities of human function there can theoretically be a different immunoglobulin for every food and/or each microbe. In reality, this does not occur. No one is allergic or sensitized to everything. What does occur is that for every food to which an individual is allergic, there is a separate, specific anti-food immunoglobulin being produced.

Just what function do these immunoglobulins perform? They actually attach themselves to—in a sense, surround—the noxious agent which could be protein, food, chemical, or microbial. This results in the formation of an *antigen-antibody complex*. These are also known as *immune complexes*. Studies have determined that in migraine sufferers immune complexes can be found in the arteries of the brain, along the brain membranes, in the arteries of the neck and scalp as well as in seemingly remote organs such as the liver, kidney, and uterus. The common medium is the blood, which transports these immune complexes and deposits them virtually everywhere. To put it simplistically the immune system will respond to improperly digested and allergic foods as if they are enemies and will launch a systemic attack. The immune complexes are one of the remnants of this attack.

In preventing allergic reactions an important element is to keep potential allergens from entering the bloodstream. One way to accomplish this is to determine a person's specific allergies so they can be avoided. However, what is most interesting is that the human body has developed its own special police force for preventing blood-borne food/chemical reactions. The key player in this force is a special immunoglobulin known as secretory IgA. It is so named because it is secreted within the intestinal tract. It is found throughout the entire intestinal canal, including the small intestine, colon, stomach, esophagus, and even the mouth. Secretory IgA (S-IgA) is produced in large quantities, some 3,000 to 5,000 milligrams being synthesized per day. This substance is highly protective against allergic toxicity. Most allergic persons secrete less S-IgA than normal, and some secrete virtually none at all.

Secretory IgA: The First Line of Defense

Secretory IgA is a critical factor in the immune defense against allergy. It is the body's initial means of defense against any toxins. What makes it the front line defender is its strategic position. Normally, this immunoglobulin is formidably poised in high concentrations along the mucous membranes of the intestinal canal. The digestive membranes are the first place where allergic reactions occur, and it is often here that significant chemical and immunological reactions develop. Reactions which occur in the bloodstream are an indication that noxious agents have penetrated the S-IgA defenses. The critical importance of S-IgA must be stressed, since it blocks the absorption of harmful substances before they gain entry into the blood or lymph. However, if noxious agents penetrate the gut, all is not lost. Internal organs, such as the liver, spleen, and lymph nodes, also contain IgA, as does the blood itself.

Secretory IgA binds to various compounds, so they can be neutralized and essentially rendered non-toxic. Also, this binding sends a signal to the immune cells, causing them to migrate to the area of the secretory IgA-bound particles. Imagine it this way: the bound particle acts as the dong of a dinner bell, as if to say, "Come and get it." This mechanism is well understood in respect to microbes, but few realize that it also occurs with allergenic food.

Imagine what would happen if a deficiency of secretory IgA existed. Virtually anything would be allowed passage from the gut into the bloodstream. Unfortunately, such deficiencies are common. Nearly one-half of Americans are lacking S-IgA, while over 70% of migraine patients suffer the deficiency. This is surely one reason so many people have migraines.

It makes sense that this deficiency is common. Secretory IgA is an immune protein. Therefore, anything which suppresses immune function negatively affects it. A wide range of substances can depress immunity and, thus, S-IgA levels. Such substances include chlorine, fluoride, solvents, heavy metals, food additives, and other chemicals. Plus, whenever a person eats an allergenic food, a certain amount of S-IgA is consumed. People continuously eat these allergenic foods. This means that those who have hidden allergies could develop an S-IgA deficiency, even if they produce adequate amounts.

Intestinal overgrowth of harmful microbes, known as pathogens, greatly impairs S-IgA synthesis. Candida albicans, a yeast, is one such pathogen. Infection by this yeast is common. The pervasiveness of this infection is ultimately a result of our antibiotic era. This is because antibiotics, whether taken as a prescription or ingested through contaminated food, selectively kill bacteria, any bacteria, that exist in the body. Billions of bacteria live in a delicate ecological niche within the human intestine. If they are killed off, as often occurs with prescription or dietary antibiotics, toxicity results. The fact is something else takes their place, and the most notorious of these is the human pathogenic yeast, Candida albicans. When overwhelming candida infection occurs, the function of immune cells throughout the body becomes severely depressed. As a result, the cells which line the digestive tract fail to reproduce adequately. Secretory IgA enhances natural defenses to prevent this yeast overgrowth. Thus, a lack of S-IgA readily leads to candida infections.

Many other factors contribute to a deficiency of this important immunoglobulin. These factors may be divided into two categories, *Diseases Associated with Reduced Levels* and *Medications Which Reduce S-IgA Levels,* which are illustrated in Tables 1 and 2.

Table 1
Diseases Associated with Reduced Secretory IgA Levels

- Crohn's Disease
- ulcerative colitis
- celiac disease/sprue
- Addison's Disease
- ataxia telangiectasia
- cancer
- food allergy
- giardiasis
- lupus
- irritable bowel syndrome
- peptic ulcer
- pernicious anemia

- chronic candidiasis
- chronic pulmonary infection
- amoebic dysentery
- cystic fibrosis
- rheumatoid arthritis
- migraine headaches
- diverticulitis
- chronic sinusitis

Table 2
Medications Which Reduce Secretory IgA Levels

- aspirin
- cortisone
- chemotherapeutic agents
- Tagamet
- Clinoril
- Pepcid
- Zantac
- Indocin
- antibiotics
- birth control pills
- Naprosyn
- antacids
- Prilosec
- Ibuprofen

From Table 1 it becomes clear that S-IgA deficiency is a common factor in many diseases, especially diseases of the digestive organs. Unfortunately, many individuals who have these diseases are taking medications, which only further accentuate the deficiency.

How can S-IgA levels be boosted? Nutritional therapy is currently the only known way. Secretory IgA is made from protein. Therefore, adequate dietary intake is important. Certain vitamins are also needed for its synthesis. Nutrients which are useful for increasing S-IgA levels include:

- vitamin A
- vitamin B-12
- vitamin C
- folic acid
- pantothenic acid
- vitamin B-6
- oil of wild oregano (P-73)
- butyric acid
- thiamine
- vitamin E

There is also the role played by intestinal health in migraines. In this regard there is a need for establishing normal intestinal health through ensuring a healthy bacterial environment. One method for this is through balancing the so-called gut. These microflora are naturally occurring bacteria which are also known as "good" or "beneficial" bacteria. There are several types, but the most common are *Lactobacillus acidophilus* and *bifidus*. Both are normal inhabitants of the human intestines. These bacteria are highly beneficial. What's more, they greatly enhance the production of secretory IgA. In other words, if such bacteria are out of balance or in decline, the synthesis of S-IgA declines significantly. The lactobacilli are readily destroyed by toxins, including chlorine and drugs. In particular, antibiotics aggressively destroy them.

Certain foods are rich in lactobacilli, including fermented milk products and other fermented foods such as sauerkraut. There are a number of top-quality acidophilus products which are available in the marketplace. One of the more sophisticated ones is the European-source Health-Bac, made by NAHS Co. The benefit of this supplement is the effectiveness in implantation. Thus, the bacteria are able to implant, that is gain residence, in the colon wall. It is ideal for traveling, since it requires no refrigeration (see Appendix C).

The human body has established numerous defenses against allergic reactions. Nature put its finest guardians on the front line. These defense mechanisms, including antibodies, especially S-IgA, protective enzymes, and white blood cells, are traumatized as a result of constant bombardment with allergenic foods and chemicals. S-IgA is particularly important, because it specifically binds toxic substances before they can cause headaches.

The measurement of secretory IgA levels in migraine patients often proves valuable. If levels are increased through natural therapies, positive results must be expected. There are no significant dietary sources of secretory IgA from foods, with the exception of mother's milk and colostrum. Therefore, internal synthesis must be relied upon to fortify this critical barrier. A strong, healthy bacterial population is one of the most effective means to achieve this. The more that is done to increase its production, the healthier the individual will become and the more resistant he/she will become to the occurrence of migraine and other illnesses.

The Leaky Gut Syndrome: A Result of Secretory IgA Deficiency?

The role of the intestines is to promote the absorption of nutrients, while prohibiting the absorption of toxins, particularly food antigens and germs. Millions of Americans suffer from a disorder where their functions are disrupted, known as the Leaky Gut Syndrome. This syndrome can be caused or aggravated by a variety of factors. Parasitic and yeast infections within the gut worsen the problem, since localized infections increase the permeability of the intestines. Such infections cause inflammation within the intestinal walls, which ultimately leads to intestinal bleeding. Prolonged infestation and inflammation may lead to significant blood loss. Thus, anemia is a common consequence of parasitic infection. The parasites damage the thin intestinal membranes, leading to blood loss. What's more, many parasites are, in fact, blood-suckers. This structural pathology leads to contamination of the bloodstream by intestinal contents, causing a sort of toxic waste leakage. Large, highly allergenic food molecules may readily pass into the bloodstream with ease. Thus, it would be no surprise that people who are afflicted with chronic parasitic or yeast infections tend to have up to twice as many food allergies as non-infected individuals.

It is virtually without exception that those afflicted with Leaky Gut Syndrome have a secretory IgA deficiency. This immunoglobulin, along with other immune defenders, helps prevent infectious organisms from gaining a foothold. Without secretory IgA, any number of noxious microbes can overgrow in the intestines. Once this occurs, they crowd out the beneficial bacteria, which only further compromises immunity, while increasing allergic tendencies.

As stated previously it was once thought that the intestinal wall is impermeable to all except the smallest molecules. Traditionally, it is taught that only the end products of digestion—amino acids, vitamins, minerals, fatty acids, and sugars—can be absorbed through the gut. According to this theory the physical barrier of the gut wall made impossible the transfer of intestinal organisms, food particles, or other large molecules into the bloodstream. This may be true of the normal mature intestine, free of disease. Yet, who has a totally normal intestine anyway?

The concept of the leaky gut was first discovered by researchers, who, to their surprise, found that up to 30% of *normal humans* absorb undigested milk proteins from a glass of milk. They also found that these symptom-free people developed measurable immune reactions to the milk proteins in the bloodstream. The reaction is called a *precipitin*, meaning that the milk protein precipitated out of solution via the phenomenon of immune complex formation.

These complexes can cause a great deal of toxicity. Such complexes could be deposited into the cerebral vessels, obstructing the circulation to the brain. In females they might end up in the uterus, causing referred pain to the head and neck. The researchers also found that the more milk that was ingested, the greater the amounts of immune complexes which were found in the blood. Yet such a reaction could occur with virtually any food, including cheese, butter, grains, eggs, meats, fish, poultry, fruits, and vegetables.

Incompletely digested food particles, as well as certain microbes, can bypass or penetrate the intestinal barrier. Even the normal intestine allows the passage of large molecules such as enzymes. The more diseased the intestines are, the more likely it is that the passage of harmful compounds will occur.

To understand how this occurs it is helpful to review human anatomy and physiology. The intestinal walls and the bloodstream are closely related. This is because it is ultimately via the circulatory system that every cell and organ is fed. Blood and lymph deliver nutrients directly to the tissues. The function of the digestive tract is to break up the food particles into a usable form. Innumerable arteries supply the digestive organs with oxygen-rich blood, and still more vessels drain wastes away from the gut. The lymphatic vessels, the "other" circulatory system, are also innumerable and are critical for assisting in the absorption of fat-soluble nutrients such as fatty acids, cholesterol, and certain vitamins. Thus, the arteries, lymphatic vessels, and veins serve to carry away and deliver nutrient-rich blood with its vitamins, minerals, fats and proteins.

It is revealing to view this at a microscopic level. The small intestine, the site where over 90% of nutrient absorption occurs, contains billions of tiny finger-like projections called *intestinal villi*. Here is where absorption ultimately takes place. The barrier between the villi and the tiny vessels which surround it is microscopically thin. Disease, inflammation, drugs, toxic chemicals, and infection all disrupt the delicate structure of the villi. So can allergic reactions. The result is a leakage of unwanted substances into the circulation. A good example of the type of damage that can occur to the delicate villi is the food allergy-related disease, *celiac sprue*. Also known as *gluten intolerance*, this disease leads to wholesale destruction of the intestinal villi. The entire absorptive surface of the small intestine can be obliterated, just from eating gluten-containing grains.

In gluten intolerance, typically, the greatest offender is wheat, although rye, oats, millet, and barley also contain gluten. Gluten is the protein portion of the grain. In this disease the immune system regards gluten as a toxin and attempts to destroy it. The immune warfare that results leads to widespread destruction of the gluten. Since gluten has a high affinity for attaching to the intestinal villi, in the conflagration these villi are often the first to be destroyed. However, the destruction is not permanent. The intestines have an astounding ability to regenerate, and the villi are ultimately "regrown." Organ tissue may also regenerate. Yet, for such repair to occur it may take weeks or months. However, the destructive cycle repeats itself, that is whenever a bit of wheat, rye, oats, or barley is eaten.

Certain nutritional supplements speed tissue repair. Such supplements include OregaMax capsules, Infla-eez, Royal Kick, the wild greens drops, and Resvitanol powder.

Anyone who reads labels knows that there is hardly a food on the supermarket shelf that is free of wheat flour, wheat germ, gluten, rye, oats, barley, malt, or similar grain derivatives. Designing a gluten-free diet is a major project. However, the improved health that results is well worth the effort.

I am gluten intolerant. I know from personal experience that one bite of bread is enough to initiate the destructive cycle. Wheat is the most commonly consumed of the gluten-containing grains, and there are millions of wheat addicts. Wheat products are cheap, convenient, and tasty. Many people find it difficult to give up wheat. Yet, those who are gluten intolerant must do so if they wish to achieve consistently good health.

Many gluten-intolerant individuals are vulnerable to developing migraines. This is partly due to the damage that occurs within the intestines. However, a more likely mechanism is what happens when antigens of incompletely digested wheat, rye, oats, or barley enter the bloodstream. Here they are attacked by the immune system. Many of these antigens are deposited in arteries of the brain, head, and neck, where massive inflammation and, therefore, pain ensue.

The allergy-prone individual can do much to protect himself and/or herself. The value of secretory IgA was mentioned. Certainly, boosting the levels of this substance would greatly help in the prevention of allergic reactions. The body has other protective mechanisms such as the liver, with its ability to clear toxins and allergins. If noxious agents enter the bloodstream, they are processed by this formidable organ. Nearly all the blood leaving the gut must first pass through the liver before it can enter the systemic circulation. The organ is well prepared for this. Structurally, the liver resembles a massive sieve. Nearly 1/3 of its mass is made up of specialized immune cells known as *Kuppfer cells*. These cells are essentially landlocked white blood cells. Thus, they act as a sort of "biological net," trapping such compounds as food antigens, bacteria, and toxic chemicals. In a sense the Kuppfer cells act as a spider web-like trap for microbes as well as allergenic proteins. Once these microbes are trapped, the Kuppfer cells begin the final kill. Ultimately, they digest the microbes, rendering them harmless.

Every day the human liver destroys billions of microbes. Thus, it can be readily understood how a sick, malfunctioning liver could predispose an individual to a wide range of illnesses. A toxic or sick liver is incapable of fully cleaning dangerous toxins or microbes from the blood. Such microbes may more readily invade the body, causing disease. What's more, the more overloaded the liver is with infection or inflammation, the less capable it is of preventing food antigens from gaining entry into the circulation. Liver diseases of all types increase the vulnerability to allergy and, therefore, migraines. A list of these diseases includes:

- cirrhosis
- hepatitis
- liver abscess
- Gilbert's disease
- Wilson's disease
- cancer
- obesity (which causes fatty liver)
- hemochromatosis (severe iron overload of the liver)
- hemosiderosis (moderate iron overload of the liver)
- Epstein-Barr syndrome

Every day the liver receives multiple doses of toxins and microbes as a consequence of what an individual eats, drinks, and breathes. People with these diseases or, for that matter, any health condition should avoid contact with substances which increase liver toxicity. These include agricultural chemicals such as insecticides, herbicides, and fungicides. The use or exposure to such substances must be strictly curtailed. They also include drugs, whether recreational or medical, and, of course, alcohol. Also, it would be important to avoid anything which weakens the gut wall and predisposes the entry of microbes into the bloodstream. This is another argument against the use of aspirin for the treatment of migraines, since it weakens the stomach and intestinal walls and causes microscopic intestinal bleeding. Other medications which aggravate the Leaky Gut Syndrome and, thus, increase the likelihood of liver toxicity include:

1. Bufferin and Excedrin
2. Indocin
3. Clinoril
8. Tanderil
9. Tolectin
10. Motrin (ibuprofen)

4. Butazoladin
5. Coumadin
6. heparin
7. Naprosyn

11. Dolobid
12. Fenoprin
13. Fiorinol
14. cortisone

Anything which increases the permeability of the gut places great pressure upon the liver. Extensive drug intake may damage the intestinal lining to such a degree that, in a sense, the flood gates are opened. Leakage of bowel contents is possible. This results in toxic reactions within the blood and internal organs and, thus, headaches. Drugs can cause a serious liver disorder called *chemical hepatitis*.

Alcohol is probably the most common and most potent offender. There is a duo mechanism by which it damages the liver; alcohol weakens the gut wall, plus it directly damages the liver. Alcohol precipitates migraines. Nearly one half of migraine sufferers are sensitive to it. The avoidance of alcohol is a must for those who wish to be cured of their migraines. Remember, one drink is enough to impair liver function. Women are particularly sensitive to alcohol's noxious effects. Regular consumption, i.e. one or two drinks per day, is sufficient to cause a certain degree of permanent liver damage in alcohol-sensitive women.

Of all alcoholic beverages wine is the primary migraine provoking drink, especially red wines. One reason is that in addition to its alcohol content wine contains several other migraine provokers. Most dominating are sulfites and tyramines. Sulfites are added as a preservative and tyramines are natural by-products of the fermentation process. The fact is tyramines are microbial by-products. What's more, they are highly toxic, especially to nerve tissue. Red wine can cause violent headaches—but so can hard liquor as will virtually any other alcoholic beverage, including beer.

Food Additives: A Major Cause of Allergic Migraines

The cause of migraines is not due exclusively to foods and beverages. There is another complicating factor: food additives. Food additives are defined as substances, whether natural or synthetic, which are added to original food sources. A good way to illustrate this concept is to consider an example of a natural unprocessed food: the cucumber. It might be presumed that a cucumber is about as natural as a food can get. However, today a cucumber is no longer just a cucumber. Fresh cucumbers contain additives in the form of waxes and coatings, which are added to enhance visual appeal as well as for preservation. A pickle is even more corrupt. Besides the garlic and dill, pickles contain up to ten different food additives. This is the challenge with nearly all the food supply. Usually, there is no way to be certain what a person is getting.

Sulfites: Culprit Number One

Sulfites are chemical agents supposedly used to prevent food spoilage. In reality, sulfites are utilized more to enhance the visual appeal of food than to preserve it.

It is well known that sulfites are toxic. This toxicity can be severe. The FDA has attributed numerous fatal allergic reactions to sulfites. Yet, it has failed to ban them as food additives. As a result, sulfites are found in a wide range of processed foods. Just inspect a few labels the next time you are in the grocery store. It is common to find the words sulfite, bisulfite, metabisulfite, sodium metabisulfite, potassium metabisulfite, and sulfur dioxide. Although originally a gas, sulfur dioxide, once ingested, can be metabolized into sulfites.

All sulfite sources are potentially toxic, causing both symptoms and allergic reactions. The degree of these reactions varies, but they can be severe enough to cause shock and death. This occurs rarely and only in highly susceptible individuals. The toxicity is usually mild, manifested by flu-like syndromes, aches, swelling, runny nose, sneezing, and, of course, headache. However, the occurrence of a single death from food additives is unacceptable. Food should create health and vitality, not illness and premature death. Yet, deaths from sulfite toxicity are far more common than the statistics indicate.

Children and adolescents are particularly vulnerable to the toxicity of sulfites. Apparently, they are less capable of detoxifying them than are adults. However, adults also may be reactive, and sulfite-induced illnesses commonly occur in them as well.

How does sulfite toxicity occur? One way is that once ingested, sulfites are transformed into *sulfur dioxide*. This is the same gas which is responsible for acid rain. Sulfur dioxide (SO2) is highly toxic. It causes damage to the lungs, immune system, and digestive tissues. Sulfites produce toxicity through another mechanism. It has been discovered that these chemicals are easily absorbed into the bloodstream and in some instances may be absorbed immediately after ingestion. Researchers have determined that there is little or no protective barrier to impair absorption once sulfites come into contact with mucous membranes or skin. This is why they are so rapidly transported into the blood. The quick absorption places severe stress on the immune system and liver, both of which are responsible for detoxifying sulfites. If the immune system and liver are overloaded, the sulfite-sensitive individual may experience a fatal or near fatal reaction. This is known as *anaphylactic shock*. This reaction is more likely to occur in a person already plagued with allergic problems or those with weakened immune systems.

Certain nutritional deficiencies also increase the vulnerability to sulfite sensitivity. Most notable are a lack of vitamin B-12 and the mineral *molybdenum*. While most people are familiar with B-12, few have heard of molybdenum. This is a trace mineral naturally found in the soil and water. It is also found in wholesome foods. However, molybdenum is highly sensitive and is easily destroyed by cooking and/or food processing. For example, the refining of whole wheat grain into white flour leads to the loss of over 80% of it. Thus, commercial foods are essentially devoid of this mineral.

It becomes easy to comprehend why molybdenum deficiency is common. What makes this mineral so important is that the key enzyme system for detoxifying sulfites is dependent upon molybdenum. In other words, without molybdenum, the enzyme becomes incapacitated. According to recent research, sulfite-sensitive individuals become more tolerant of sulfites if molybdenum is supplemented in the diet.

B-12 also assists in the detoxification of sulfites. Its value is greatest during a sulfite reaction, as supplemental B-12 has been shown to minimize the severity of the reaction. How much B-12 should be given? As much as 1000 micrograms three times daily during and for a few days after the reaction is the recommended anti-sulfite dose.

Sulfite Toxicity and Restaurant Food

Most of the publicity concerning sulfites and sulfite sensitivity has revolved around the use of these chemicals in restaurants. Here, careless or misinformed workers often add excessive amounts of sulfites to foods as a preservative. Uninformed workers may fail to measure the proper amount, adding several times the needed amount.

Sulfites are used in an attempt to preserve visual quality and prevent oxidation. Oxidation is the process by which foods become discolored or brown. Foods which typically receive a sulfite bath include lettuce, fresh vegetables, fresh cut potatoes, fish, shrimp, and fruit. Here is a rule to go by: If such foods are on a restaurant menu, they contain sulfites until proven otherwise. If there is any doubt, it is always a good idea to ask. However, many servers are unaware of how sulfites are used and have no knowledge that severe toxicity can occur. Ideally, have the server ask the food preparer or the chef if sulfites are used.

A neglected area as a source of sulfites is the grocery store, or perhaps it should be called the "additive store." The latter is an accurate description. Virtually every packaged food has a potentially noxious additive. Since most grocery store items are either canned, jarred or boxed, it is accurate to say that over 90% of the items in the typical grocery store contain one or more food additives capable of causing allergic reactions. Sulfites are among the most pervasive. Many are aware that dried fruits, beer, and wine contain sulfites. A partial list of other foods and beverages containing sulfites includes:

- jarred fruits
- fruit drinks
- fruit salads
- salads (deli)
- diced melon and/or other deli fruits
- fruit toppings and fillings
- jams and jellies
- sugar (brown or white)
- gelatin
- bakery
- pie fillings
- tortilla chips
- soups, especially canned
- French fries and Tater Tots
- relishes
- pickles
- olives
- salad dressings
- potato salad
- guacamole
- gravies and sauces
- canned vegetables
- frozen vegetables (some)

- poptarts
- pancake mixes
- pancake syrup
- batters and breading
- cornstarch
- potato chips

- vinegars
- coffee
- instant tea
- breakfast drinks
- hard liquor
- TV dinners

Is this a list of prohibitions? It is for the sulfite-sensitive individual. Yet, in general if the objective is to achieve improved health, then most of these foods should be avoided.

Hundreds of drugs contain sulfites. Especially suspect are drugs which are inhaled or injected. Many oral drugs also contain sulfites. These include heart medications, steroids, antibiotics, pain medicines, and muscle relaxants. This is bizarre, since many such drugs are given precisely to treat the symptoms caused by sulfites. There should be a public outcry over the use of sulfites in drugs and foods. They serve no useful purpose and, rather, cause great harm.

MSG: Culprit Number Two

MSG, monosodium glutamate, is a synthetic food additive. Rather than serving any nutritional value it is used to create heightened taste sensations. Like sulfites, MSG is in a huge percentage of commercial foods. It also is used extensively in restaurants, especially oriental ones. MSG is used simply to enhance flavor. It has no known nutritional value.

MSG is such a noxious compound. It is a toxic chemical, and let it be stated so, lest there be any doubt.

Some researchers classify MSG as a *neurotoxin*. A neurotoxin is defined as a substance, whether natural or artificial, which exerts powerful toxicity upon the nerves and may cause permanent nerve damage. There is another dangerous side to MSG: It is a drug. So says George Schwartz M.D., author of the provocative book, *In Bad Taste: The MSG Syndrome*. If you find this hard to comprehend, that a drug could be allowed to be liberally added to food, you might want to read this informative book. Turn to page 16, where this brilliant scientist calls MSG, "a poison," and pages 19 and 121, where he proclaims it to be a drug. According to Dr. Schwartz MSG is found in most foods—everything from fried chicken to hamburger meat—and in a majority of packaged foods found in the supermarket. Numerous research studies on MSG are quoted in his book. Among the findings are:

- Over twenty million Americans are highly sensitive to MSG, while nearly one third exhibit a lesser degree of sensitivity.
- Symptoms range from mild reactions to serious ones requiring hospitalization.
- If the dose is high enough, everyone will react to MSG.
- Children are highly sensitive to MSG, and chronic exposure may result in behavioral disorders or impaired intellect.
- Brain damage is possible if the dose is high enough and the usage is prolonged.
- MSG consumption may be associated with neurological diseases including Lou Gehrig's disease, Alzheimer's disease, and Parkinson's disease.

More Than Just the "Chinese Restaurant Syndrome"

Many people believe that the only way to get an MSG reaction is to eat at a Chinese restaurant which loads up its food with MSG. This is untrue. MSG is used heavily by virtually all fast food restaurants. Wherever there is breading, there is also MSG.

Breadings and butter are used extensively in fast foods. There are Chicken McNuggets and Kentucky Fried Chicken.

There is Popeye's, Churches, and Brown's fried chicken and Wendy's chicken sandwich. There are fish sandwiches, tenderloins, cheese balls, fried zucchini, onion rings, and breaded mushrooms. There are veal and eggplant Parmesan, breaded pork chops, chicken fried steak, and many other grease-filled and MSG-coated foods. These greasy and MSG-tainted foods are toxic and may cause a wide range of symptoms. Ultimately, the ingestion of such toxic foods results in diseases such as heart disease, digestive disorders, and cancer.

You can get the Chinese Restaurant Syndrome at virtually any restaurant, even in fine dining establishments. Have you ever heard of Lawry's seasoning or Accent? Both contain as their active ingredient, MSG. The seasonings are commonly used in fine dining restaurants to flavor meats and vegetables. Thus, MSG intoxication should be renamed the "Fast Food and/or Fine Dining Restaurant Syndrome."

There should be an additional syndrome. It is the "Grocery Store MSG Syndrome." Every supermarket in this country has foods on its shelves which are laced with this insidious substance. MSG has infiltrated virtually every grocery store shelf, and nearly every product contains either "MSG," "hydrolyzed vegetable protein," "autolized yeast," "hydrolyzed yeast," "vegetable powder," or "natural flavors" all of which are an indication of added MSG. It's unbelievable. When you read labels at the grocery store, you discover that a huge percentage of food contains it. It's as if we cannot live without it. MSG has so polluted our taste buds that most people would not know what food tastes like without it.

Is it anything but sensible to presume that canned tuna, especially tuna packed in "spring water," is completely natural? It isn't, since it probably contains MSG. How about dry-roasted nuts? They are supposedly all-natural. However, many brands are laced with MSG. What about fresh meats? Some stores add MSG to "enhance flavor." How about frozen vegetables? Those which have sauces usually contain MSG. It has gotten so maddening that it would be easier to make a grocery-store list of foods without MSG than to list those which contain it. The next time you go to the grocery store search for yourself. Surely you'll find this to be true, and you'll be astonished, if not appalled, at the number and variety of foods which contain this chemical.

The major difficulty in determining the presence of MSG in foods is that it can be disguised by other names. An extremely common one used by food processors is "natural flavors." This is found in many foods, including ketchup, soups, cured meats, canned meats, noodle/pasta dishes, and frozen dinners. While it cannot be stated with certainty that MSG is included as one of these natural flavors, its presence is more likely than not. This suggests that even many of the foods labeled "all natural" may not be entirely safe.

Migraine-like headaches are one of the two most common symptoms associated with MSG sensitivity, the other being a "tight feeling around the face or neck." The MSG headache can be mild, moderate, or severe. What's most problematic is that the headache often occurs hours or even days after the time of ingestion. Thus, it may be difficult to trace the cause of the headache. On the other hand, some people react almost immediately. Other symptoms associated with MSG sensitivity include:

- chest pain or pressure
- depression
- diarrhea
- dizziness
- eye pain, eye irritation or blurry vision
- fatigue
- heartburn
- hot flashes

- insomnia
- nausea
- numbness around the face
- pain radiating down the arms
- palpitations
- sore throat
- stomach cramps
- sweating
- urinary discomfort

Admittedly, it is not easy to eliminate all exposure to MSG. However, every effort should be made to limit exposure, especially if there is a history of migraines. While some people are allergic to MSG, everyone is sensitive to it. This is because MSG is truly a toxic chemical, one that everyone should avoid.

Food Dyes: Culprit Number Three

Thanks largely to the work of Dr. Feingold, a medical doctor, whose research came to light in the 1970s, many Americans have become aware that food dyes are bad for the health. Early research correlated the ingestion of artificial colorings (dyes) with learning disorders. A new disease called childhood hyperactivity, now known as attention deficit disorder (ADD), was discovered at about the same time. Children with this disorder were so hyperactive that they were unable to concentrate at school. Often they were placed in lower grades or special classes; many were drugged with Ritalin. This practice is continuing today.

What is less commonly known is that food dyes cause migraines. How these noxious compounds were ever allowed into the food supply remains an enigma. Food dyes are highly toxic chemicals. Most are known carcinogens. Yet, Americans continue to consume several tons of food dyes every year. Regarding migraines probably the greatest culprit is Yellow Dye #5. Ironically, its chemical structure is nearly identical to that of aspirin. In fact, it is classified chemically as an aspirin derivative, i.e. a salicylate. This means that people who are allergic to aspirin are also allergic to the dye. Another name for Yellow Dye #5 is *tartrazine*, and it may be so listed on food labels.

Yellow Dye #5 is a common ingredient in packaged or canned foods. It is found extensively in fast foods, ice cream, and candies. A partial list of foods or substances containing this dye includes:

- pickles
- relishes
- prepared salads
- canned fruit
- butter
- cheese
- margarine
- frostings
- puddings
- hard candies
- popsicles
- ice cream
- Kool-Aid
- gelatins
- colored cereals
- lime flavoring
- Gatorade
- banana flavoring
- sherbet
- mustards (some)
- Mountain Dew
- rum
- apple and cherry turnovers
- pop tarts
- children's cereals
- wine coolers
- drugs
- multiple vitamins
- orange, yellow, or light green fruit drinks
- baked goods, especially those with yellow creamy puddings
- soft candies—yellow, orange, or light green in color.
- hot dog/hamburger buns, especially those with yellowish tint

Through a mechanism similar to sulfites Yellow Dye #5 also can cause allergic shock. This usually occurs in highly allergic individuals, such as asthmatics, who are allergic to the dye. It rarely occurs in migraine patients, since their allergies result from a different mechanism. However, this serves to demonstrate how incredibly toxic the dye can be.

There are numerous other common food additives, far more than can be listed. Several thousand are approved for adding into the food. The majority are synthetic chemicals devoid of nutritional value. Most are petrochemical derivatives or by-products of coal tar. Such derivatives are proven carcinogens. Thus, as far as human health is concerned, such substances serve no useful purpose. The internal chemistry of the human body—the functioning of our cells and organs—has no need for food additives. The nutritional value of a substance should be the standard upon which decisions are made concerning what is and isn't allowed into the food supply. The American public must strive to get the more toxic additives pulled off the market and out of the foods. Some of the more common food additives *known to cause allergic reactions* include:

- NutraSweet
- sodium benzoate
- saccharin
- artificial flavors
- caramel color
- octylgallate
- carrageenin
- sulfites
- dextrin
- shellacs and waxes
- dextrose
- caffeine
- artificial colors
- propylene glycol
- propylgallate
- MSG
- sorbitol
- hydrolyzed yeast protein (contains MSG)

Both synthetic and natural food additives can cause allergic reactions. Few of the synthetic additives have undergone careful enough scrutiny to be labeled "unequivocally safe." Allergic reactions are not the only debacle. The fact is chemical additives are a major cause of cancer. This is serious business. Toxic chemicals are inappropriate for food. Every effort must be made to have them removed from the food before further death and decimation occur. Some of the better known cancer-causing chemicals, which, incredibly, can be legally added to food are listed below:

- coal tar derivatives (food dyes, artificial flavors)
- acetaldehyde (a nerve and brain toxin)
- propylene glycol (a component of antifreeze)
- chlorine dioxide (toxic chlorine gas, a known poison to the lungs and intestines)
- butane (lighter fluid)

This is just a small list of the many toxic chemicals which are found in our food or used in food processing. The addition of these carcinogens to food should never have been allowed. What is most puzzling is how a supposedly educated, health conscious nation could allow such blatant negligence to occur and to continue to occur. When will the people, for the sake of personal health and that of the future generations, stand up against this crime?

Make no mistake about it, antifreeze is inedible. It is toxic, even in the tiniest amount. It belongs in an automobile, not in the human body. The challenge is yours, to speak out against this crime now or wait until it is too late. Do write the food processors. Your efforts will be recognized. A good example is the butter industry. This industry is ultra sensitive to consumer pressure. Land O' Lakes of Minnesota is now in the forefront, having replaced the carcinogenic coal tar dye *Butter Yellow* with the non-toxic natural dye, *annato*. Buy Land O' Lakes butter (or, preferably, organic butter), and let the industry know that natural is the only option and that certainly it is the consumer preference. Believe me, the rest of the butter manufacturers and possibly the margarine producers will soon follow suit. The result will be that butter dyes made from cancer-causing substances will become obsolete.

Food Additives and the Migraine Patient

For the migraine sufferer the point is simple: processed foods, packaged foods, shelf foods, and fast foods are far more likely to provoke headaches than natural unaltered ones. The definition of a natural food is one to which *absolutely nothing is added; no flavor enhancers, no invisible antioxidants, no food colorings, preservatives, emulsifiers or stabilizers.* Just plain clean fresh food—this is the safest to rely upon.

Eating in restaurants can be a significant hazard for the migraineur. The reason is that there is no way to be certain regarding what is in the food. In most restaurants, food is heavily laced with additives. Some fine dining restaurants may be the exceptions. Since many of these restaurants make their food from scratch, it is easier to specify changes in the menu. Most of these restaurateurs are willing to accommodate individual health needs. Just tell them that you could have a serious allergic reaction, and watch the response. Few servers are skilled at CPR. Plus, such servers are scared of the liability. Isn't pain, severe pain, a serious symptom? Don't be shy to take whatever steps are necessary to ensure that the things you are sensitive to are kept out of the food. Remember, you are the one paying for the service, and you will be the one who will pay the price if a severe migraine strikes.

Of course, fast food restaurants are the worst of all. It would be impossible to list all the additives typically found in fast foods. Such foods are loaded with grease, hydrogenated oils, food dyes, MSG, sulfites, artificial flavors, nitrites, sugar, corn syrup, milk, white flour, white rice, starch derivatives, NutraSweet, caffeine, caramel color, and salt. The majority of these substances can instigate headaches. The real danger is when several such additives are combined at once. This "additive" effect can lead to a headache severe enough to last for days. Simply look at commercial food labels. It becomes readily apparent how common it is to ingest foods with a large number of additives. Some foods contain dozens of synthetic chemicals. Thus, certainly, processed foods are a major cause of toxic reactions, including migraines.

Despite all this it is possible to eat out and do so safely. Any restaurant which is willing to cook fresh foods from scratch—organic meats, poultry, seafood, fish, and vegetables as well as fresh fruit—would be acceptable. In this regard it is possible to get a meal occasionally at certain fast food restaurants, although organic meat is hard to find. Yet, it doesn't cost much more to eat at a nice restaurant. A meal at a fast food establishment can cost as much as $12.00 to $20.00, which is not much less than the price of a basic meal which can be purchased at many supper clubs. By the time the aspirin or Tylenol is added to deal with the consequences, a person would nearly break even.

Real Food: The Major Cause of Migraines

Up to now the discussion has been primarily about how chemicals, toxins, synthetics, fumes, and food additives can cause headaches. Could foods by themselves be as insidious in generating migraine headaches? They are, and, incredibly, they cause far more migraines than do chemicals or food additives.

There are several mechanisms by which foods cause migraines. No two migraine patients are alike in terms of how they react to a given food. Plus, each person has developed his/her own specific set of food allergies. True, there are some foods which are highly likely to provoke migraines. The list usually includes coffee, wine, cocoa, tea, eggs, wheat, and cheese. While it is true that many migraine patients are allergic to these foods and beverages, a significant number are not. Those who are not necessarily allergic to the typical triggers are often allergic to various other foods or additives—ones which are rarely suspected. Such foods are equally potent in causing migraines. For this reason it is difficult to make a comprehensive list of foods to avoid. In the typical diet there are several hundred common foods, beverages, and additives. No list could be comprehensive and also be specific. Even so, the following is a list of the more common foods which, through testing and clinical experience, have been found to be common migraine provokers:

- cocoa
- coffee
- eggs
- wheat
- sulfites
- food dyes
- barley

- MSG
- cheese
- orange
- tobacco
- wine
- corn

Mechanisms of Food Allergy: Migraine Reactions

This is mentioned, because the thinking in the scientific community for years has been that the protein part of the food is a major initiator of allergic reactions. Many of the aforementioned foods contain little or no protein. Yet, they commonly trigger allergic migraines. It is now known that allergic reactions can be caused by a variety of other compounds. In fact, non-protein allergic mechanisms probably cause just as many migraines if not more than do those initiated by proteins. Let's look at some examples.

Potatoes contain protein, but they are primarily a starchy food. A common allergic reaction to potatoes results from a contaminant found on the skin, an alkaloid produced by a fungus that grows on potato skins. Neither starch nor protein is involved. This contaminant is extremely toxic, as is manifested by the severe headaches it causes.

Wine contains no measurable amount of protein. Yet, headaches which result from the drinking of wine are both common and severe. Wine contains *amines*, a kind of modified amino acid (not a protein), plus sulfites, mold residues, etc. These amines have an aggressive biological action. They are toxins produced by the microbe, which ferment starches and sugars. As has been previously mentioned, wine aggravates allergic tendencies by another mechanism: it increases the permeability of the intestinal wall, allowing easier passage of potentially toxic compounds into the bloodstream. Alcohol is a solvent, which causes tissue damage. The delicate tissues of the human intestines are exceptionally vulnerable to its toxic effects. It has a direct toxicity to both the stomach and intestinal walls. In addition, people can become sensitized to the original source of their favorite drinks: grapes in the case of wine; malt, yeast, and hops in the case of beer, and grains in the case of liquor.

Lemons and limes contain aldehydes, citrus oils, and flavonoids, all of which can provoke headaches. Even the smell of a freshly cut lemon can cause a headache in certain highly sensitive individuals. A minimal exposure can cause maximum pain. Cocoa contains *theobromines,* which are chemically related to caffeine. Theobromines have direct toxicity upon the nervous system. Caffeine also operates via this mechanism.

Wheat contains a protein known as gluten. This protein by itself can generate migraines. It also contains highly reactive compounds known as *neuroactive peptides.* These compounds exert a direct poisonous effect upon the brain. Neuroactive peptides, in fact, bind to brain cell membranes at certain receptor sites, notably the receptors for insulin. This is disastrous. Here, these chemicals prevent insulin from its normal function, which is assisting the entry of glucose into brain cells. Thus, the brain is unable to retrieve sufficient amounts of glucose from the blood, and the energy deprivation results in a headache.

If protein antigens enter the bloodstream, that's when the real trouble begins. A wide range of immunological and chemical reactions directed against the antigens are likely to occur. Commonly, the result is inflammation, nerve irritation, clogged circulation, and reduced oxygen supply. Pain is inevitable.

These inflammatory reactions can develop locally within pain sensitive regions of the head and neck. Or, they can occur in distant sites, causing the phenomenon of referred pain.

During the menstrual period allergy-induced inflammation within the uterus, fallopian tubes, or ovaries can result in migraines. Here, toxins or allergens can directly irritate the female organs, provoking migraines. Similarly, an allergic reaction occurring within the stomach, liver, or intestines can lead to head pain. Long term damage: an ominous result.

When toxic allergic reactions develop within the cranium, the result can be quite severe. The constant inflammation due to migraines can weaken the involved tissues. Recently, researchers discovered that long term migraine sufferers are at risk for a serious condition known as dissecting cervical and/or cranial arteries. This means that the arteries of the upper neck and also those within the skull may spontaneously split, leak, or even burst. When an allergic migraine occurs, the arteries, especially the smaller ones, become inflamed. If this happens repeatedly over a prolonged period, scarring and other damage may result. With time, this process weakens the arterial wall, increasing the risks for serious disorders, including strokes.

There is an additional factor the researchers failed to consider. Most chronic migraine sufferers take heavy doses of aspirin and/or similar drugs. It is likely that this drug consumption plays an even more critical role in weakening the blood vessel walls than the allergic reactions. Nutritional deficiencies also contribute to arterial disease. Often, such deficiencies are induced by drugs. Vitamin C is critical for the formation of collagen, the protein which keeps the arteries glued together. Heavy doses of aspirin, meaning more than three aspirin per day, decimate tissue vitamin C levels. Aspirin also destroys folic acid, another nutrient needed to maintain strong arteries.

Thus, it becomes readily apparent why excessive aspirin consumption is one of the major causes of spontaneous brain hemorrhage. Indocin, a drug commonly given to arthritics and gout patients, also compromises vitamin C and folic acid levels.

The fact is all anti-inflammatory drugs destroy this vitamin. Those taking cortisone rapidly become vitamin C deficient. Cortisone also destroys other B-complex vitamins. Other nutrients necessary for keeping the arteries strong which are compromised by drug therapy include vitamin E, vitamin A, vitamin K, and bioflavonoids. Here, a natural vitamin C and bioflavonoid supplement could prove invaluable. Natural vitamin C is far more effective in strengthening blood vessel walls than the synthetic. Flavin-C is a natural vitamin C supplement containing vitamin C only derived from fruit and wild herbs.

Recently, an astonishing medical finding was reported regarding the damaging effect of chronic migraines. Many migraine patients suffer a visual disorder: they, in fact suffer a loss of their peripheral vision. Although the visual loss is mild, it does indicate that damage is occurring. The likely cause? Impairment of circulation to the retina due to the destruction of tiny retinal arteries and veins or damage resulting from the toxicity of pain medications.

All this is merely another reminder that it is of the utmost importance to either eliminate the migraines or reduce their severity. Ideally, this should be accomplished without further compromising health with potentially toxic medications. It defeats the purpose to treat the symptoms with medicines which worsen the underlying conditions. Doing everything possible to help relieve the pain is important. Getting to the bottom of the cause and striving to cure the migraine condition is mandatory.

Can Food Allergies Short-Circuit the Brain?

Food allergies cause physical symptoms. Pain is one of those symptoms. Yet, could mental symptoms result from food allergies? Rarely do people directly associate eating a specific food with mental or psychological symptoms. It is now known that allergies can cause mental aberrations. Using a sophisticated neurological test, researchers have found a way to prove that what we eat affects our brains. They actually measured toxic allergic reactions while they occurred within the brain. Let's see how this fascinating story evolved.

Decades ago researchers found that certain chemicals irritate the nervous system. Most notable of these is the pesticide DDT. It was found that the chemicals, even in very small doses, damaged the nervous system, often permanently. The brain and spinal cord were most vulnerable to this damage.

These experiments were conducted with a device known as an EMG or electromyograph. *Electro* indicates electricity, *myo* is Greek for muscle and the term *graph* is self-explanatory. Thus, an EMG is the measurement of electrical activity within muscle tissue, which is plotted via a graph. This test is performed by placing electrodes in the patient's muscle tissue, the muscles are stimulated using a small amount of electrical current. Under normal conditions when a muscle is stimulated, a certain level of activity is expected, and this activity is represented by the height of the spikes on the graph. When researchers exposed subjects to DDT, the height of the spikes dropped measurably. In addition, these persons developed pronounced symptoms, including poor coordination, weakness, slumping of posture, blurry vision, drowsiness, and even the feeling of being confused or stupid. Other substances which were found to depress the EMG included synthetic perfumes and cigarette smoke.

The most astounding discovery was that food, in this case the common hen's egg, could have a similar effect. A 39-year old woman was the subject of the study. Her primary problem was migraine headaches, which she developed after a severe viral infection. She also complained of problems with coordination and muscular weaknesses. An EMG was performed by first testing her muscles in the normal state to get a baseline. Then, she was fed two scrambled eggs. Within an hour she became ill. Her hands trembled, her speech was slurred, her posture slumped and her legs weakened. She became uncoordinated, and her muscles began twitching. At this point the EMG measured greater than a 50% reduction in muscle activity and strength. All this was due to a food allergy. Similar defects occurred after food challenges with her other migraine-provoking foods, which included milk, chicken, and shrimp.

Fortunately, it is unnecessary for headache sufferers to undergo such a painful ordeal as having electrodes implanted into the muscles. Yet, this does illustrate a point. Certain foods and chemicals have a direct and potent influence on brain and nerve function. All nerves arise from the brain. Nerve-related symptoms, whether painful or psychological in nature, often have a physical component. Only rarely is pain or neurological disease primarily psychological in origin. With regard to migraines it is important to always assume that the pain is physical, not mental.

Do Children Have Migraines?

This brings us to an important subject: children. They often complain of "hurt" or pain. Children can develop headaches, even at very young ages. Allergic headaches may occur as early as 2 or 3 years of age. What is most interesting is the way they describe their headache pain. Children don't understand what constitutes a headache. All they know is that they hurt. In fact, children with migraines often fail to relate that they have head pain and may complain of seemingly unrelated symptoms such as a tummy ache. This becomes a problem, since many parents and doctors disregard the child's complaints as being largely psychological. In this regard a common thought is that the child is complaining in order to get attention or "love."

Presumably, children have better things to do than to complain about pain. If a child says he/she is in pain, it should be regarded as true until proven otherwise. In fact, an effort should be made to be sure the pain is not due to a serious problem. It should never be written off as "psychological." Believe me, most children would rather be playing in a sand box, digging holes in the ground, playing with toys, watching cartoons, making mud pies, coloring, or performing some other enjoyable endeavor than complaining about how much they hurt. When a child says he or she has a sore throat, we listen attentively and believe. Why not pay attention when other complaints are expressed? Migraines are common in children, and they occur more frequently as children age. The teenage years are a time when migraines often begin, and during this time they can be severe. As the immune system matures the frequency of headaches due to food and chemical sensitivity increases. When the immune system reaches its pinnacle, as in adulthood, the incidence of migraines also reaches its zenith.

So, when a child says he/she has pain in the head, even if at a tender, young age, do pay attention. That child may well be developing the beginnings of an allergic migraine. If this condition is diagnosed early enough, a great deal of suffering can be prevented, not to mention problems such as aspirin, codeine, and other drug dependencies.

There is a challenge in diagnosing allergy-induced migraines in the very young. Their allergies change with time. Plus, blood tests are usually ineffective. It is difficult to make the diagnosis via laboratory testing, because the immune system of these youngsters is so immature that measurable reactions against foods are limited. Instead, one must attempt to establish the diagnosis through trial and error and then avoid the suspect foods. Once a child reaches age 9 or 10, accurate testing can be performed. For information on such testing call 1-800-243-5242. Substances which commonly provoke headaches in this age group include:

- MSG
- peanuts
- sugar
- corn syrup
- cocoa
- cola nut
- alcohol
- salicylates
- corn
- wheat
- cow's milk
- brewer's yeast
- cheese
- NutraSweet
- eggs
- soy
- food dyes
- baker's yeast
- nitrated meats (bologna, salami, ham, etc.)

In general, children have horrible eating habits. Much of their diet consists of foods which are nutritionally inadequate. What market do the sugar-coated cereal, ice cream, and candy manufacturers target? Who are the primary consumers of candies, cookies, popsicles, soda, candy bars, chips, and other junk foods? What group do the fast food chains target? The answer is obvious. Fully overwhelmed, children readily succumb to marketing hype and stand no chance of defending themselves. They are true victims of a system, which is ruthless.

Children are targeted for financial reasons, never their health. This is criminal. The fact is they are constantly eating and drinking food which should be classified as nutritional garbage. The consequences are disastrous. Diet-induced health problems in children are exceedingly common. The incidence of juvenile diabetes is increasing dramatically, as are diseases such as obesity, high cholesterol, and cancer. In what is a frightening trend children are dying young from diet-induced diseases, including heart attacks, sudden death, allergic shock, and cancer. Such diseases were virtually unknown in children as little as 70 years ago. Yet, it is not merely the physical disease which results. A wide range of mental diseases in children are directly due to sugar ingestion. This substance is a fulminate poison. It is unfit for human consumption. It is particularly unfit for children. What's more, it readily destroys the developing brain. This is why a wide range of mental symptoms and diseases, including hostile behavior, mood swings, attention deficit, autism, depression, and anxiety are directly tied to sugar consumption. Even truancy and poor scholastic performance are connected. For your children significantly reduce the consumption of all forms of refined sugar. As a result, you will help them avoid long-term health crises. Sugar destroys the internal organs, including the brain. Its destructive effects are unforgiving. Refined sugar is ruining the lives of our children. Do not knowingly participate in this debacle by encouraging the consumption of this poison.

What can be done about this? A great deal, if parents take the initiative. Remember one thing. Addicted children can have one of two main reactions; they either can be worn down or hyped up by a high sugar, junk food diet. The hyped up ones are especially tough customers to cure. This is particularly true in the early stages when attempts are first made to get them off this junk food, a stage more commonly known as withdrawal. That's right, these children are addicts. Whatever the efforts might be, the benefits are well worth eradicating their addictions. It is up to parents to take charge of the situation and get the kids off addictive, nutritionally depleted foods. They may well develop into pussy cats as a result and become easier to control in terms of their eating habits. The benefits can be fascinating: improved grades, better behavior, less mood swings/temper tantrums, and, most important, improved health.

Believe it or not, some people actually give their children wine and/or beer to drink and think it is funny. This is far from a joke and must be regarded as a dangerous practice. Alcohol is a common cause of migraines, and so are the chemicals (e.g.

sulfites, preservatives, etc.) it contains. Worse, even small amounts can cause learning disorders and brain damage in youngsters. This vulnerability is partly a result of the immaturity of the nervous system. The brain cells are just beginning to develop and are growing at a very rapid rate. This means that the nervous systems of children are far more susceptible to the damaging effects of alcohol than are adults' nervous systems, which are fully matured. Plus, children can become physically and psychologically addicted to alcoholic beverages much more easily during the teen or adult years if they become accustomed to "booze" early in life.

It is unlikely that people who do this to children give thought to the potentially disastrous effects, ultimately, but they should. They must carefully consider the implications of what they are doing: alcoholism, drug dependency, mental disorders, and chronic illness are all potential results. Maybe those who do this have brain damage themselves from "pickling" their cerebral cortex with alcohol or drugs.

Alcohol can turn an adult into a child, because it destroys the brain's vitality, rendering brain cells useless. It is an unpleasant thing to see, but it is very real. On the other hand, alcohol in no way makes a child more mature. If people took heed of this, this nation would be a better place to live for all. Alcoholism leads to the destruction of everything from the home to the human body. It is a 100% minus. Even the alcohol industry is urging moderation. Let's do our best to keep alcoholism at bay by keeping alcohol out of the mouths of our babies.

White and Dangerous: Artificial Sweeteners, Major Headache Promoters

Since the turn of the century white powders have become a fixture of American culture. There are hundreds of white powders. Some are chemicals, others are drugs and still others are actual foods. Cocaine is a white powder, and so is aspirin. Sugar is white. Naturally brown whole wheat flour is bleached until it becomes as white as a sheet.

White implies clean. Beautiful white linen symbolizes cleanliness and prepares us for our meal. White paper towels and tissue paper give us a clean feeling when we use them. It doesn't seem to matter how these products become white. That white toiletries, cloths, and powders contain residues of bleach and dioxin, both of which are toxic, seems to make no difference. What matters is that they are white. After all, who would think of cleaning the kitchen with unbleached, environmentally safe, brown gritty looking paper towels? We need white to be clean.

The food industry and the industrial community are aware of this mentality. They are constantly working in their labs to find new, magical white substances: enter the artificial sweeteners. Of course, these too are white powders. The other white powder, sugar, is still heavily consumed. Much of this sugar consumption is in the form of "hidden" sugar. Ketchup, which is nearly one third sugar, is a good example.

How does sugar become white? It is bleached with chlorine or bromine gas to form perfectly white granulated or powdered sugar. Thus, it is processed until nothing of value remains. Artificial sweeteners are not always white as a result of bleaching. They are chemical powders made synthetically in a lab, and, like many other synthetics such as drugs, they are naturally white.

Does the fact that a substance is white really mean it is safe? Cocaine is white, but it is hardly safe. So is heroin and, the ultimate in white drug refinement, crack. White does not automatically imply safety. On the contrary, any white powder must be deemed toxic until proven otherwise. Glaringly white powders or other white substances are a signal to stay away at the risk of damaging one's health. Crisco is white, and so is lard. Insecticides, herbicides, and coal tar derivatives, such as dioxin, all are white. So when you think of white, instead of thinking of "clean," picture a skull and crossbones. What a switch in thought that would be.

The primary artificial sweeteners available on the market are NutraSweet and saccharin. Both are produced synthetically, and neither is found in nature. Both were discovered accidentally by chemists, who were working on other laboratory projects. Neither has been proven safe. In fact, much evidence exists proving highly toxic effects.

The pancreas is an internal organ which is particularly vulnerable to the toxicity of NutraSweet and saccharin. Research has shown that both of these chemicals impair the secretion of pancreatic enzymes. Even small amounts, such as that found in a single can of pop, measurably reduces enzyme levels. Pancreatic enzymes are of vital importance. Without them, food cannot be properly digested. The toxicity of incompletely digested food has already been discussed.

There is an additional means by which these agents cause migraines: direct chemical toxicity. This is especially true of NutraSweet, a well known cause of migraine. NutraSweet can act as a nerve toxin, exerting ill effects upon the brain. In fact, there are several cases on record of NutraSweet-induced neurological disorders, and it has caused both reversible and irreversible visual loss.

All these effects are thought to be mediated within the brain by a highly toxic by-product of NutraSweet metabolism: *methanol*. This substance is also known as *wood alcohol*. In even modest amounts methanol causes blindness and death. A mere tablespoon is enough to kill, virtually immediately. A vile poison, Hughe's textbook of medicine describes it as the most potent of all poisons. Some 10% of the weight of, for instance, a packet of NutraSweet consists of methanol. No wonder NutraSweet consumption leads to neurological disorders and provokes migraines.

NutraSweet, known by the chemical name aspartame, is a potent neurotoxin. It consists of methanol bound to two different amino acids. Once it is digested, the methanol is released. This methanol is quickly absorbed into the blood. From here it readily penetrates nerve tissue, where it causes massive damage. Methanol is a solvent. It strips the lining of nerve tissue, exposing it to the elements. This makes the nerve sheath highly vulnerable to disease and infection. It also interferes with key enzymes within the nerves, including those which control critical functions such as breathing and the pumping of the heart. This is why methanol is such a deadly poison.

People consume NutraSweet as if it is of no consequence. Yet, they have no clue of its toxic nature. Regular consumption greatly increases the risks for permanent nerve damage. The nerves most vulnerable to its toxicity include those which control vision, taste, and hearing. NutraSweet is also toxic to the internal organs, particularly the liver and pancreas. The regular use may lead to significant damage of such organs. Symptoms of NutraSweet, that is aspartame, intoxication include dizziness, sinus problems, headaches, migraines, bloating, indigestion, bad taste in the mouth, burning or sore tongue, canker sores, confusion, visual disturbances, spots before the eyes, blindness, hearing loss, and seizures.

It is a crime to put such a deadly poison in food. The fact is the perpetrators of such a crime must be held to account.

Saccharin also exerts direct toxicity to the nerves, but it is a less common cause of migraine than NutraSweet. One only wonders what other "sweet" white powders will be legalized for dumping into food. If the FDA won't regulate these substances more carefully, who will?

Your Fillings: Can You Be Allergic to Them?

Metal allergy is relatively common. Medical allergists, as well as dermatologists, are aware of this phenomenon. One of the most common metal allergies is to nickel, a component of jewelry. This allergy usually manifests itself as a skin rash at the point of contact such as under a watch or beneath a necklace. Yet, can a person actually be allergic to his/her own fillings? It is possible, since fillings are also made of metal, but a different type. Most people have silver fillings or, more correctly, silver-mercury fillings. These fillings provoke allergy reactions and headaches.

The correct terminology for the common silver filling is *dental amalgam of the silver-mercury type.* In reality these fillings are a combination of many metals and, thus, may also contain nickel, tin, zinc, and other materials. Gold fillings also contain several minerals, but these fillings are less common and rarely cause illness.

Most people, when having their cavities filled with silver-mercury amalgams, thought that the material being placed in their mouths was harmless. They had full trust in the dental professionals that they would certainly have studied amalgam to ensure it is non-toxic. Unfortunately, no such thorough studies were ever performed. The fact is that over one-half the weight of these fillings consists of mercury, one of the most toxic elements known.

Mercury is best described as a *neurotoxin*, meaning it is highly toxic to the nerves. Of all nerve tissue the brain appears to be the most susceptible. Apparently, mercury has a predilection for deposition in the type of fat found in the brain. It simply dissolves directly in it. Here is a story that is significant. In the 1920s and 30s, top hats were popular. These hats contained an inner band that was lined with mercury. The mercury was absorbed from the bands through the facial skin and scalp into the blood and then deposited in the brain. People who worked in the hat factories handling and installing the linings were known as "mad hatters." Back then, no one had any idea why they were crazy. Now, it is known that it was the mercury that was responsible.

For over the 100 years that dental amalgam has been placed in teeth the people have been led to believe that the practice was entirely safe. Those who questioned the logic of putting mercury in the mouth were told that metal amalgams were inherently stable and that the mercury would stay in the filling forever with no chance of leaking out. Yet, modern science has proven this theory was erroneous. Dental amalgams leak mercury, and this leakage is detectable. Measurable amounts of mercury from dental fillings can be found in the blood, liver, kidneys, nerve tissues, and hair of individuals with silver-mercury fillings.

Who is to blame for this madness? Must the dental profession be held responsible? These are difficult questions, and there are no simple answers. However, dental professionals should be the first to issue warnings concerning the dangers of dental amalgam. Instead, the public is reassured that no such danger exists. The fact is the dental profession spends millions of dollars trying to prove that amalgam is the only reliable source for quick, effective fillings. If only a fraction of these dollars were spent in a positive way trying to find an alternative to amalgam, it would be quickly developed, and this public menace would finally be eliminated. Possibly, the dental profession to their surprise would find a public willing to make any concession if it meant less danger and better health.

The informed public wants this dangerous practice stopped. If the dental profession only knew how much was at stake, maybe it would be driven to positive action instead of wasting time making excuses.

There are several ways that amalgam provokes headaches. Being a direct neurotoxin, it weakens nerve tissue, increasing the risk for chronic pain and migraine. It is possible to be allergic to the metals in the fillings, and this can lead to headaches. An even more powerful mechanism involves electrical currents. Metals conduct electricity. What has only recently been appreciated is that when metal is in the mouth, it readily conducts electricity, especially if several metals exist simultaneously. The saliva acts as the conducting medium, and the fillings act as charged poles. This electrical current is most pronounced when silver and gold fillings are found together in the mouth. It seems that this creates vulnerability to a certain type of migraine induced by biological electrical currents.

The dangers of mercury absorption into human tissues can no longer be denied. While many people are allergic to nickel or tin, nearly everyone is allergic to mercury. It is truly a universal toxin and, be assured, if it exists in the mouth, it is leaking and contaminating tissues and organs throughout the body. For instance, a team of researchers in Calgary, Alberta, found that dental amalgam in the typical doses to which humans are exposed causes kidney damage. The researchers placed amalgam fillings in sheep. Shortly afterwards the sheep developed kidney damage manifested by a measurable loss of kidney function, whereas the kidneys of the control sheep remained normal. Their conclusion: Dental amalgam should be banned immediately.

There is yet another sinister effect of mercury toxicity: immune decay. Mercury destroys immune cells. Immune cells are responsible for absorbing any remnants of mercury found in the tissues and, thus, bear the brunt of the injury. With a weakened immunity and a damaged nervous system, it is easy to see how something as seemingly unrelated as silver–mercury fillings can be a primary cause of headaches.

I was first alerted to this connection as a medical student by a wonderful lady named Mary. She had the problem of daily or near daily migraines. Nothing seemed to help her. Megadoses of vitamins and minerals were virtually useless. Osteopathic manipulative treatments were regularly performed with only minimal relief. Acupuncture proved fruitless. Trigger point injections did little more than provide temporary relief. Finally, Mary went to a dentist knowledgeable about the problems of "modern" dental fillings. He immediately determined the problem. Not only did Mary have silver-mercury fillings, but she had gold ones as well. The dentist felt that the two different metals resulted in the formation of an electrical current in the mouth. He was right: all metal fillings were extracted, and Mary's headaches greatly improved. Remember, nothing else relieved her headaches, that is until the fillings were removed.

For those who have amalgam fillings there are thousands of dentists throughout the country who believe in the toxicity of mercury and are willing to carefully extract this poison. Dentists themselves are well aware of the dangers of mercury. When raw mercury is first mixed with other metals to form amalgam, the dentist and/or technician must handle the substance with great care. The fumes from the mercury are so toxic that they can be fatal. Special warnings on the in-office handling of mercury are issued by the American Dental Association. Masks and gloves must be worn. Yet, this noxious compound is and has been freely placed in human mouths for decades.

The migraine sufferer should seriously consider having amalgam fillings removed. Adequate replacement fillings are available. Be sure to search for a competent, qualified dentist, who understands the problems of mercury fillings and can lead you through this.

When considering the toxicity of mercury, is it any wonder that dentists have the highest suicide rate of any profession? This is surely due to the ill effects of their exposure to mercury. This mercury is the prime cause of the depression and suicidal tendencies commonly seen in dentists as well as dental technicians. One study in a prominent medical journal, *The Lancet*, showed that dentists have extremely high levels of mercury in their brains and that the pituitary gland is particularly vulnerable. Mercury levels in the dentists' pituitary glands were up to 100 times greater than normal. The connection to suicide becomes obvious. The pituitary controls the hormone system, and hormones control mood. A dentist with depression, agitation, anger, anxiety, and suicidal ideation surely has mercury overload of the brain.

Mercury poisoning is a serious dilemma and, as previously mentioned, can lead to kidney damage, immune system diseases and neurological disorders. Symptoms of mercury intoxication include insomnia, memory loss, agitation, mood swings, headaches, anxiety, bleeding gums, depression, bad breath, and tremors. Those who have mercury/silver fillings and are concerned about toxicity may wish to contact the office of Dr. Hal Huggins to obtain more information and a referral to an Alliance Dentist specifically trained for this purpose. For more information, please call (toll-free) 1-866-948-4638.

Food Allergies and Migraine: Selected Case Histories

When a migraine sufferer has his/her allergies diagnosed and when an appropriate treatment regimen is applied the results are predictable: there will always be improvement. It is helpful to read about real life examples. The following pages describe several examples of migraine cures. Yet, anyone who is plagued with headaches could gain the same results.

So read on. The cure is available for all who pursue this effective approach.

Lemon allergy the cause of horrible migraines

Ms K. is a wonderful lady whose expertise is in the field of preventive health care. She fought a long standing battle with debilitating migraines and tried everything she knew for relief. The migraines, occurring as often as five times per week, were severe enough to keep her bedridden and unable to work. Her work was very important to her, and she tried everything to eliminate the headaches, often resorting to consuming as many as 20 to 30 aspirin a day in an attempt to control the pain. Since she had read that allergies could be involved, she attempted to discover her allergies through the time consuming method of food elimination, withdrawing foods and reintroducing them, as a means of determining the causative foods.

As is commonly the case with health care professionals, Ms K. was resistant to the idea that she had additional hidden food allergies and that these were the likely cause of her headaches. I advised her that this was probable, but she said, "I already know what my allergies are." I insisted that she had no scientific way of knowing, and finally she relented and the Food Intolerance Test was performed. The results showed a severe citrus allergy as well as allergies to butter, pork, kidney beans, filet of sole, scallops, walnuts, apples, malt, nectarines, tobacco, cashews, coffee, and mint. Incredibly, every day she squeezed a wedge of lemon into her water under the impression that this was good for digestion. While it may be a digestive aid for persons who are not allergic to it, lemon in water is a digestive disaster for those who are. Lemon contains a variety of natural chemicals, which can provoke migraines. In Ms K.'s case, removing the lemon alone eliminated over 70% of her headaches. Most of her other headaches were caused by mint, malt, pork, coffee, and tobacco. Just being in a room filled with tobacco smoke was enough to provoke an immediate headache.

Severe tobacco allergy is common and is found particularly in smokers and ex-smokers. The most likely cause of headache in smokers is the tobacco they smoke. Part of their addiction may well be a result of their tobacco allergy. Ms K., a former smoker, is now headache free, that is unless she eats one of her allergic foods or is exposed to tobacco smoke.

25 years of migraines eliminated literally overnight

Mr. D. experienced headaches usually on a daily basis. Although Mr. D. consulted several doctors, the cause was never determined. Sophisticated tests, including CAT and brain scans, as well as an MRI, failed to determine the cause.

By the time Mr. D. had arrived at my office, he had long since given up on finding any cure for his headaches. In fact, he came to see me for an entirely unrelated problem. Since his symptoms indicated the existence of food allergies, testing was performed. Mr. D. was found to be extremely sensitive to wheat, so sensitive that a diagnosis of *celiac disease or gluten intolerance* was established. Gluten is the protein found in wheat and certain other grains including oats, barley, millet, and rye. As described previously wheat contains proteins called neuropeptides which are irritants to nerve and brain tissues. In people who are severely sensitive to wheat, even a tiny amount can provoke symptoms.

Mr. D. had been eating whole wheat products daily for years, though he had rarely eaten white flour. He had done this because he was under the impression that "whole wheat is good for you." His perception was understandable. Unfortunately, despite the fact that whole wheat is a natural food, in his case no wheat is the only policy to follow. Wheat and all foods containing wheat flour, bran, or germ were removed from his diet.

Since wheat is in most processed foods Mr. D.'s diet was rather limited. However, the extra discipline was worth it. By eliminating wheat he also got rid of his daily headaches.

As it turned out Mr. D. was a wheat addict. He ate pasta and/or bread daily. He is not alone. There are millions of wheat addicts. For some of these addicts wheat or foods containing wheat, such as cereals, crackers, and bread, make up over 50% of the diet. Here is a rule of thumb. Wheat addicts who have headaches are probably allergic to wheat, and wheat allergy is the likely cause of their headaches. Other foods or substances may be involved such as baker's yeast, which is added to all commercial crackers, pastries, buns, and breads. However, in my experience the wheat proteins found in wheat flour, whether from white or whole wheat, cause a greater amount of headaches than all the additives combined.

Migraines so severe that she pounded her head against the wall

Ms J.'s migraines were both frequent and intense. At times the pain was so agonizing that she pounded her head against the wall, or on a table or desk. Somehow, she insisted, this gave her temporary relief. Allergy testing revealed over 20 foods to which she was sensitive. After eliminating these foods, the headaches gradually dissipated. However, to attain more complete relief, neck injuries resulting from a car accident were treated with OMT and trigger point injections (see Chapter Six). Ms J.'s headaches have improved over 60%, although treatment is continuing. Her allergy profile is as follows:

- scallops
- crab
- egg
- molasses
- corn

- cola
- cashews
- dill
- sardine
- lobster

- cheddar cheese
- soy bean
- peanuts
- walnut
- cocoa/chocolate

- shrimp
- oyster
- pork
- mustard

Mother of two with weekly migraines allergic to all American staple foods

Mrs. B.'s migraines were frequent and severe. Each attack lasted over 48 hours. At times they were so intense that she stayed in bed for the duration of the pain. Mrs. B.'s diet was heavy in the American staples including milk products, eggs, citrus, and wheat. Oranges, orange juice, and wheat bread were her favorite foods. Her allergies included the following:

- egg yolk
- pork
- butter
- wheat
- orange
- peanuts
- kidney beans
- sulfites

- pinto beans
- walnuts
- cashews
- cottonseed oil
- margarine
- saccharin
- cola

Mrs. B. experienced a dramatic improvement in her headaches, and as long as she avoids her allergenic foods, she is headache-free. Her quality of life has improved dramatically. She is happier, thinks more clearly, and has more energy than she's had in years.

Any one of the aforementioned foods or substances can trigger headaches. The problem is that many commercial foods contain several of these items, and this is an exponential danger for headache sufferers. For example, consider deep fried fish. The fish is preserved with sulfites, and the breading contains wheat, cottonseed oil, non-fat milk, and margarine. Plus, it is deep fried in more margarine, cottonseed oil, and/ or lard. For Mrs. B. a fried fish sandwich would amount to consuming five allergenic components in the final product. A severe migraine would likely result.

Killer headaches due to wheat/rye allergies

Mrs. Z. experienced severe migraine headaches on almost a daily basis. Often developing suddenly, the headaches were so intense that they forced her to leave work. Mrs. Z. was a senior receptionist in a doctor's office. Two trips to Mayo Clinic and one to the Diamond Headache Center proved fruitless. Through specialized testing it was determined that she had a chronic intestinal yeast infection, but, more importantly, it was also found that she was highly allergic to wheat, wheat bran, rye, and cheese. Removal of the allergenic foods and treatment of the yeast infection led to a dramatic improvement. Mrs. Z. is now headache-free for the first time in 30 years, as long as she stays away from wheat and rye.

Severe secretory IgA deficiency related to migraines

Mrs. G.'s migraines were unusually severe. When they occurred, she became debilitated for up to three days. A week did not go by without some type of headache afflicting her. Each one was different. Sometimes they were accompanied by nausea. At other times they were associated with visual disturbances and eye pain.

Testing determined she had a deficiency of secretory IgA. Thus, she had minimal protection against allergy reactions. Mrs. G. had an allergy to limes, lemons, cocoa, butter, cheddar cheese, mozzarella cheese, nectarines, apples, English walnuts, mint, and black walnuts.

Treatment included allergy removal and nutritional therapy to increase the secretory IgA levels. A multiple spice capsule, known as Migraten, was also added. Today, she is headache-free.

Sinus headache due to milk products

Mrs. H. had a history of headaches which occurred primarily in the front of her face. This area is commonly known as the sinus region, and, technically, her headaches were more sinus-type migraine. For over 20 years she experienced headaches which occurred as often as twice a week. Also, she complained of a chronic problem with stuffy sinuses and postnasal drip. However, there was another peculiar complaint: she occasionally vomited after eating, even though she had no nausea or pain. This symptom in particular was highly suspect as being food allergy in origin.

In susceptible people food allergy reactions can lead to a phenomenon known as *pylorospasm*. The pylorus is a muscle or, to be more specific, a sphincter located where the stomach ends and the intestines begin. It controls the rate at which stomach contents are emptied into the intestines. In Mrs. H.'s case allergenic foods greatly irritated the nerves of the stomach which control the sphincter. The pyloric spasm was so violent that vomiting ultimately resulted. Her primary allergies were as follows:

- cocoa
- milk
- butter
- cheese
- corn
- sugar
- molasses

Mrs. H. related that the vomiting commonly occurred after eating her favorite late night snack. As might be suspected this snack contained nearly all these substances. It was a chocolate bar and a glass of milk, a snack which often ended up in the sink. After she quit consuming this addictive snack the vomiting and headaches disappeared. She also had relief from her sinus congestion, which was likely a result of the sugar and milk allergies.

Forty year old realtor allergic to junk foods and sugar

Mr. W. had no idea why he had migraines nearly every day. He noted that stress made them worse, so he assumed this was the primary cause. Upon inquiry, it was determined that allergies were the likely culprit. His horrible diet was loaded with junk foods, sweets, and fast foods. A typical breakfast consisted of doughnuts and coffee. He frequently ate deep fried foods such as French fries and fried chicken. Cookies and sweet rolls were his favorite snacks.

It was no surprise that Mr. W. was allergic to many of the ingredients commonly found in these foods. His allergies were as follows:

• molasses	• cheddar cheese
• sugar	• mozzarella cheese
• maple syrup	• yeast
• corn	• MSG
• corn syrup	• saccharin
• beef	• margarine (cottonseed oil)
• fish	

Mr. W. was unaware that he consumed a daily dose of most of his allergenic foods, and this was the cause of his migraine. MSG is found in virtually every fast and processed food as are yeast derivatives, sugar, molasses, and corn syrup. Beef and cheese are primary components of pizza, burgers, and other fast foods. Margarine is used in the majority of deep frying fats. Doughnuts, sweet rolls, breads, cookies, chips, and fast foods all contain margarine or other types of shortening. Mr. W.'s headaches disappeared within four weeks, since he strictly adhered to his new diet. This was a fantastic result for a man who thought his headaches were due to the "unavoidable" stresses of his job.

Administrator of nursing school relieved of migraines

Susan J., an R.N., had suffered with migraines for over 15 years. She tried many orthodox therapies over the years, but nothing seemed to help. She became resigned to living with the pain. After hearing me speak on the radio, she decided to investigate the allergy approach.

Susan's migraines were classical. They were usually preceded by visual disturbances and often accompanied with nausea. The nausea was most bothersome and, like the headaches, lasted for days. Susan had an unusually high pain tolerance, so she took no medicine for the headaches. She had to "tough it out," since her job was important to her. She was not about to let the pain inhibit her.

Food allergy was the primary cause of Susan's symptoms. She also had a severe case of chronic candidiasis secondary to antibiotic toxicity, and this illness increased the allergic tendency. Her allergies were as follows:

Severe	Moderate
• egg	• shrimp
• butter	• lobster
• lamb	• pork
• tobacco	• mozzarella cheese
• dill seed	• sugar
• walnuts	• molasses
• sulfites	• soybean
• cinnamon	• salicylates

Note the allergies to chemicals and chemically treated foods. Soybeans, molasses, and seafood usually contain residues of toxic chemicals, particularly pesticides and herbicides. This sensitivity shows a significant degree of adrenal exhaustion. Thus, in addition to eliminating the allergenic foods adrenal supplementation is necessary. She was given adrenal-boosting formulas, for instance, AdrenoAid, as well as pantothenic acid. As a result of the elimination of food allergies, as well as supporting adrenal function, Susan is now free of headache pain for the first time in 15 years.

Talk show host for news radio station is allergic to the foods of his own state

Jan is a respected talk show host for the #1 news radio station in Iowa. I appeared on his show numerous times. He claimed he was healthy, but this was obviously untrue. Like nearly all other media personalities, he had highly destructive eating habits and constantly ate junk and fast foods. While on the air I pressed Jan about his faulty eating habits. He admitted to having memory problems, lags in concentration, and occasional bouts of fatigue, especially after eating. These are cardinal symptoms of food intolerance. The pop, chip, and pizza man consented to a food allergy test.

The test was performed and the results were playfully discussed on the air. These results proved that allergies were the major problem: he had over 40 of them. They included pork, beef, butter, cheese, corn, cane sugar, and cola. Jan is originally from Iowa, and, as I told him over the air, he is allergic to it. The major farm products of Iowa include corn, pork, beef, and milk products.

Jan had never complained of headaches. Yet, after the allergies were diagnosed, and he avoided his most addictive allergy foods, headache was the first symptom he noticed when cheating. He noted on the air that after eating a bag of corn chips, he got a "splitting headache." When he religiously avoids the allergenic foods, he is headache-free. Now, Jan is a true believer in the migraine-food allergy connection.

Took so many medications you would expect her to rattle

Mrs. R. experienced some of the most severe migraines conceivable. She had all the classical symptoms: nausea, visual disturbances including loss of peripheral vision, one-sided pain, throbbing pain, etc.

Due to the severity of the pain Mrs. R. resorted to medication. During her 25-year battle with migraines she consumed literally thousands of pills, including aspirin, Tylenol, Advil, Sine-Aid, and Excedrin. There were times when she had taken aspirin "by the handful."

Mrs. R.'s migraines were partly allergic and partly structural in origin. Allergy removal, manipulative treatment, and trigger point therapy all were employed. Migraten was also provided at a dose of two capsules daily. The results were astounding. The frequency of headaches was reduced from five or six per week to less than one per month if any. Plus, when they do occur, they are far less severe and last only a few hours rather than days. The fact is Migraten, with its potent content of anti-inflammatory spice extracts, helped obliterate her headaches.

Haven't heard that laugh in years. . .

Pamela, a 32-year old mother of three, experienced daily headaches. She originally developed them as a freshman in college, and they worsened with time. Toward the end of college she was diagnosed by an internist as having "migraine phenomena."

Pamela's headache pain was debilitating. She found little or no relief in medication. Doctors told her nothing could be done; she was informed that she was "high strung" and also a "worrier." These comments affected her greatly, and she began to feel "responsible" for her headaches. Guilt developed, and so did depression. Yet, she always remained hopeful for a cure and minimized the intake of addictive medicines as much as possible, with the belief that one day she would conquer the headaches.

When I saw Pamela, her lifestyle was poor. Her daily headaches were of low-grade intensity, and she could count on at least one severe migraine each week. Minor stresses and seemingly insignificant problems could result in a mind-bending headache. It was all she could do to get the kids dressed, fed, and ready for school. Then, she would lie down and turn off the lights to hide from the pain. Allergy testing revealed Pamela was allergic to several foods which she commonly consumed, including eggs, pork, beef, butter, cane sugar, corn, cheddar cheese, beans, asparagus, and cocoa. Through a combination of osteopathic manipulative treatments, allergy elimination, and trigger point injections, Pamela is now headache-free. That is why her sister observed such a monumental change in her that she said, "I haven't heard you laugh like that in years."

Summary

Allergies are a major cause of migraines, but there are many other factors as well. Yet, there is little doubt that allergies to foods are the number one factor. To pursue the allergy approach is to open the door to what will likely lead to a new life, one free of pain. If you are a migraine sufferer take that chance. It will be well worth it.

Chapter 5

Hormonal Disorders: The Number Two Cause

Hormones are closely tied to the occurrence of migraine. Tension or stress headaches may be hormone related, since stress or tension damages the glands, particularly the adrenals. Women who have PMS migraines are well aware that their hormonal cycles are closely tied to headaches. Headaches related to drops in blood sugar levels are also hormonally induced, since hormones, such as cortisone and insulin, control blood sugar levels. Migraines are the primary hormonally induced headaches.

There are several types of hormones. Virtually all hormones are produced by specialized glands known as *endocrine glands*. These glands control a vast array of functions, including digestion, heart rate, protein metabolism, body temperature, sexual capacity, fertility, blood sugar regulation, and uncountable others.

Brain Cells Control Our Hormones

The brain is the ultimate power behind the hormone system. Within it are two extremely important segments or glands, the *hypothalamus* and the *pituitary*. The pituitary is a true gland, while the hypothalamus is essentially a section of brain tissue. As the hierarchy goes, the brain or cerebral cortex, that is the thinking portion of our brain, controls the hypothalamus. The hypothalamus exerts direct control over the pituitary. The pituitary fully controls the rest of the hormone glands.

Through these interconnections our thoughts and moods have a direct effect upon the synthesis, secretion, and function of hormones. So does stress, which greatly upsets their chemistry. Also these organs, the brain, hypothalamus, and pituitary, must respond to the survival needs of the body. These are known as involuntary functions and include the rhythmic beating of the heart, breathing, blood vessel tone, digestion, and nerve conduction.

The pituitary is a tiny gland about the size of a pea. However, its size is no representation of its importance. This critical gland sends special hormonal messages to all other endocrine glands, signaling when to make, or when to stop making, hormones. It also communicates to them what type of hormones to make. In this way the pituitary controls the function of the pancreas, liver, thymus, adrenals, ovaries, testes, and thyroid.

When the pituitary is stressed, headaches can result. One way this occurs is through the phenomenon known as *hypertrophy*. The term is defined as an increase in the size of an organ secondary to excessive cell growth. This essentially means that the pituitary is swollen. People who are under emotional stress or who have faulty dietary habits are likely to develop pituitary hypertrophy.

The pituitary gland lies within the cranium in a tight space known as the sella tursica. Often, with migraine patients doctors view x-rays for evidence of swollen pituitary glands, which can be easily defined in this restricted region. As stated in *Harrison's Textbook of Internal Medicine*, "Enlargement . . . is frequently encountered in routine skull series [x-rays] obtained in patients complaining of headaches. . ."

The swelling places pressure on nerves in the cranium, resulting in pain. The sella tursica is a weak area in the bony structure of the skull. With pressure it allows for a certain degree of give. However, many thousands of nerve fibers lie on the membranes surrounding this region. The swollen pituitary may place undue pressure upon these nerves or upon the brain itself, leading to headache. This may also lead to pain behind the eye, a classical symptom of pituitary enlargement or strain.

The pituitary keeps the adrenal and thyroid glands functioning properly. If these glands are weakened, the pituitary is forced to overwork, which leads to the hypertrophy, in other words, swelling. Thus, it is important to cure all glandular defects in order to have a healthy pituitary and in order to prevent pituitary swelling.

People whose migraines are manifested by *pain behind the eyes* almost assuredly have swollen, overworked pituitary glands. Anatomically, the gland is very close to the eyes, and this is one reason the pain is referred there. What's more, the optic nerve lies exceedingly close to this gland.

Besides the pituitary the most important glands involved in migraine are the adrenals and the thyroid. While the pituitary exerts control over these glands, the thyroid and adrenal glands secrete the most powerful hormones in terms of overall effects upon body functions. The sex glands are also important, but when compared to the role played by the thyroid and adrenals, their relationship to the cause of migraine is insignificant.

Hypothyroidism

Hypothyroidism is defined as a reduction in the function of the thyroid gland. This usually occurs to the degree that signs and symptoms occur. Migraines are one of the most common of these symptoms. Thus, when evaluating patients with chronic headaches, hypothyroidism is a major factor to consider. The precise reason the thyroid is so often involved in migraine is unknown. However, it is most likely related to the metabolic rate. The lowered metabolism in hypothyroidism disrupts the neurons, leading to swelling, inflammation, and therefore, pain. Plus, the lowered metabolism reduces the flow of oxygen in the brain, which also leads to pain.

There is another condition which results from hypothyroidism: stasis of body fluids. This can even affect the bloodstream. In the brain the circulation stalls to a virtual halt. Toxins accumulate and the oxygen levels drop. As a result, headaches develop.

Hypothyroidism should be a major consideration, especially in females whose migraines occur prior to or during menses. The thyroid is involved in the metabolism of estrogens and other sex hormones. Hormone metabolism within the liver, including the breakdown of toxic forms of estrogen, is thyroid-dependent. Defective thyroid function causes an imbalance in the hormone system such that symptoms, including PMS, hot flashes, and migraines, frequently result.

These symptoms often miraculously disappear after the administration of thyroid extract. The potency and quality of the extract, which is a prescription drug, may vary. Synthetic thyroid compounds have little if any anti-headache effect. Synthroid is the name for the typical synthetic thyroid prescription. Standardized raw (all-natural) thyroid extract is more effective in blocking and/or preventing headaches. This extract is made from the thyroid glands of animals. However, it is made from the glands of commercial cattle, which due to the mad cow epidemic has raised concerns. Yet, there is a less risky option which is available.

The thyroid can also be naturally boosted—without animal products. This is done through certain herbs, nutrients, and particularly, wild kelp. ThyroAid is a high quality combination of thyroid-boosting herbs, amino acids, and kelp. The kelp in ThyroAid is the highest quality available, free of heavy metal residues. Commercial kelp must be avoided, since it is contaminated with toxic metals, especially arsenic. Whether high or low, ThyroAid readily balances thyroid, leading to a reduction and elimination of headaches.

Women are the primary victims afflicted with hypothyroidism. It can also occur in children, teenagers, and adult males. In fact, it is reasonable to presume that nearly every American has a thyroid problem. To many such a statement might appear controversial. Let me explain. To be more specific anyone who has subsisted over a number of years on the standard American diet has an improperly functioning thyroid. This is also true of the majority of vegans and vegetarians. For the majority the diagnosis of hypothyroidism applies. Some have such a mild case that it is never noticed. Others have it more severely.

Why isn't this disorder diagnosed more frequently? Because in the majority of instances blood tests will largely be negative. Yet, the hypothyroid state exists, and the signs and symptoms are there. Hundreds of doctors and many scientists are aware that hypothyroidism can occur despite normal blood studies.

The fact is blood tests only demonstrate the abnormality in the extreme. It takes up to a 70% loss in function before blood tests are positive. Thus, for the majority a sort of undiagnosed or "sub-clinical" form of hypothyroidism is the norm. This latter form can be diagnosed largely through symptom analysis.

It is a significant claim to state that nearly every American has a thyroid problem. Some people will find this hard to believe. Many physicians will be antagonistic to the concept. However, there is a great deal of circumstantial, as well as factual, evidence upon which this argument is based. Recent research indicates that at least ten million Americans have hypothyroidism to the degree that it can be diagnosed medically. In Canada the condition is pandemic, with some 5 million Canadians affected. The thyroid gland is among the most metabolically active of all organs. It is highly sensitive to defects in nutrition. If even a single nutrient is deficient it will malfunction, let alone a whole group of them. For instance, vitamin A deficiency leads to impaired thyroid hormone synthesis as does a deficiency of zinc, copper, selenium, thiamine, vitamin B-6, vitamin B-2, or folic acid. Most Americans are deficient in these nutrients.

In a minority of instances malfunction can mean aberrant or accelerated function, and this occurs in a disease known as *hyperthyroidism*. In this condition the thyroid gland essentially burns itself out. Hyperthyroidism is treated medically with powerful drugs such as radioactive iodine. However, the use of nutritional agents such as vitamin A, natural iodine, niacin, and thiamine, as well as the highly biologically active ThyroAid, can also help alleviate the hyperthyroid condition. The niacin and thiamine can be procured through NutriSense, a drink mix rich in natural-source B-vitamins. These large doses provide nearly 50% of the RDA for these vitamins. Vitamin A can be consumed by eating fatty fish, egg yolks, and liver. The iodine is found in table salt, unbleached sea salt, red meat, and seafood. Due to its rapid rate of metabolism, the thyroid gland consumes a significant amount of nutrients. Nutritional deficiencies which directly impair its function include:

- cobalt
- coenzyme Q10
- copper
- essential fatty acids
- selenium
- thiamine
- tyrosine
- vitamin B-6

- folic acid
- iodine
- magnesium
- niacin
- riboflavin

- vitamin B-12
- vitamin C
- vitamin E

Virtually every major nutrient is needed for optimal function of this gland. Since most Americans are deficient in one or more of these nutrients, it makes sense that nearly everyone has a thyroid defect of some sort. While it is true that nutritional supplements stimulate thyroid function, in severe cases the most important element of treatment is medication: thyroid hormone. Only doctors can prescribe this compound. Testing of thyroid function both prior to and after taking thyroid hormone is advised. However, one must be aware that the tests may all be negative, and a thyroid defect can still exist. In these instances a simple at home test known as the *underarm temperature test* may prove useful. Otherwise, a trial of thyroid hormone followed by a re-evaluation of the symptoms may help establish the diagnosis.

As mentioned previously, underarm temperature can be a clue to the existence of hypothyroidism. The lower the temperature readings, the more significant are the results. This test was first developed by Broda Barnes, M.D. He found that readings consistently below 97.6 degrees Fahrenheit indicated the existence of hypothyroidism. In this instance the sluggish thyroid could no longer sustain a normal metabolic rate. The result was reduced body temperature.

Here is how this test is performed. Simply place by the bedside a standard thermometer, which has been shaken down. Upon awakening immediately place the thermometer under the arm, and don't move. Stay in bed for 10 minutes, and record the temperature. Do this for seven to ten days. Then, take an average. During this time women who menstruate often find that the temperature changes dramatically.

What does this have to do with headaches? Migraines are common in people with hypothyroidism. Some of these individuals get headaches which never seem to go away. Patients who have continuous headaches should be thoroughly evaluated for thyroid disorders. In fact, the prolonged, endless headache is what the author describes as the *hypothyroid headache*. If the more serious causes have been ruled out, anyone who has a daily headache which lasts for weeks or months must be suspected as being hypothyroid in addition to being allergic to foods. Can it be imagined—a continuous, year-long migraine? In hypothyroidism it is possible. No one knows for sure why this occurs. It seems likely that the lowered body temperature and the resulting impaired metabolism make the hypothyroid individual more vulnerable to migraine attacks. Yet, it may be simply due to a reduction of oxygen metabolism in the brain.

Many symptoms are associated with hypothyroidism. Thus, this condition can mimic other illnesses. To help solidify the diagnosis a questionnaire has been devised listing signs and symptoms which are commonly found in the hypothyroid patient. To determine your score answer yes or no to the following:

Hypothyroid Questionnaire

	Yes	No
1. Do you experience constant lethargy or weakness?	☐	☐
2. Are you tired in the morning and more energetic at night?	☐	☐
3. Do you have dry or coarse hair and/or skin?	☐	☐
4. Is your speech slowed, or do you have slurred speech?	☐	☐

5. Do you have swelling of the face and/or eye lids? ☐ ☐
6. Are your hands and feet cold? ☐ ☐
7. Do you experience bloating and indigestion after eating? ☐ ☐
8. Do you have hair loss from the outer third of your eyebrows? ☐ ☐
9. Do you have short-term memory loss? ☐ ☐
10. Do you experience depression, which is worse in the winter or on overcast days? ☐ ☐
11. Do you have white spots on your fingernails? ☐ ☐
12. Do you have chronic weight problems? ☐ ☐
13. Are you easily constipated? ☐ ☐
14. Do you experience PMS and/or menstrual disorders? ☐ ☐
15. Do your feet or ankles swell? ☐ ☐
16. Do your hands swell? ☐ ☐
17. Do you have chronic headaches? ☐ ☐
18. Are you emotionally unstable? ☐ ☐
19. Are your nails brittle? ☐ ☐
20. Do you exhibit lack of sweating? ☐ ☐
21. Do you have a poor appetite or a lack of hunger? ☐ ☐
22. Are you generally nervous? ☐ ☐
23. Do you have pale skin? ☐ ☐
24. Do you have a dry throat, or do you experience hoarseness? ☐ ☐
25. Do you have hair loss (particularly females)? ☐ ☐
26. Do you have a difficult time getting deep breaths? ☐ ☐
27. Do you experience heart palpitations? ☐ ☐
28. Do you have severe muscle cramps? ☐ ☐
29. Do you bruise easily? ☐ ☐
30. Do you have joint stiffness? ☐ ☐

Add up the number of positive answers. If you answered up to 5 as yes, the diagnosis of hypothyroidism is possible. If you answered between 6 to 11 positively, the diagnosis is virtually assured. If 12 to 19 were positive, the diagnosis is certain. A score over 20 indicates a severe case of hypothyroidism.

If you have headaches and there is evidence that you are hypothyroid, rest assured of one fact: if the thyroid condition is properly treated, the headaches will improve. In fact, they may well disappear altogether.

The Thyroid Gland and Circulation

Previously, it was mentioned that migraine headaches occurring over a prolonged period can lead to damage of the arteries in the head and neck. Obviously, migraine is, to some degree, a vascular disease.

The thyroid gland exerts significant control over the circulatory system, and this is one reason disorders of this gland are related to migraine. Thyroid hormones act directly upon the heart and are responsible for increasing its pumping power, that is its ability to move blood through the circulatory system. Also, thyroid hormones exert powerful control over heart rate, either increasing or decreasing it. Furthermore, the tone of the arteries is dependent upon this hormone.

It has long been known that people with hypothyroidism often have elevated cholesterol and triglyceride levels. Broda Barnes, M.D., has repeatedly demonstrated that hypothyroid patients are at a significantly increased risk for developing heart disease. The low metabolic rate and reduced carbohydrate metabolism probably account for the increased levels of blood fats, but what accounts for the higher incidence of heart attacks observed in this group? It is likely due to this fact: hypothyroid patients tend to have unhealthy arteries. The more severe the thyroid dysfunction, the worse the arteries will likely be.

Diseased arteries cause enormous strain on the heart. Arteries are supposed to be soft and flexible, making it much easier for the heart to pump blood through them. However, when the arteries harden, a condition known as *atherosclerosis*, the heart must pump extra hard to force blood through such arteries. Plus, the arteries supplying the heart itself can become hard, which is known as *coronary atherosclerosis*. This further impairs cardiac function by reducing blood flow to the heart muscle itself. The term *sclerosis* indicates a scarring and hardening of the tissues often complicated by the deposition of calcium. Thus, the relevance of arterial diseases to migraines is clear. Poor circulation, with resultant reduced blood supply to the brain, increases the risk for migraines. Plus, if the arteries of the brain are themselves diseased, the connection becomes even clearer. Thus, in order to cure or prevent migraines the health of the arterial system must be improved. Proper balancing of thyroid function through improved nutrition and the intake of ThyroAid will greatly help in this regard.

There is another circulatory mechanism linking hypothyroidism to migraines. As may be recalled the thyroid gland is regarded as the "master of metabolism." This relatively small gland controls the metabolic rate for every organ and function. In hypothyroidism everything is slowed. Another way of comprehending this is to use the term "depression." In the hypothyroid individual every physical and mental function is depressed. Blood flow is reduced, as is evidenced by symptoms such as cold hands and feet, dizziness, palpitations, etc. However, a measurable depression of cardiac function, in terms of clinical disease, only occurs in extreme cases of the disease.

A good analogy of the ill effects of decreased thyroid function is how the pistons of an engine pump when a car is started in freezing weather. The thick oil causes the pistons to move sluggishly until the entire engine warms up. With the hypothyroid individual the engine never completely warms up. As a result, a sort of sludging of the blood occurs, and, thus, circulation to the end organs is decreased. This accounts for many of the symptoms seen in hypothyroidism, especially cold hands and feet.

Few solutions are offered to hypothyroid patients. They just keep plugging along with their sluggish disposition, depressed manner, fatigued and sluggish or apathetic personality and, often, with their frequent headaches. They try everything to rid themselves of their health problems—some even resorting to psychiatry—but nothing provides any lasting relief.

Such patients are often given sedatives and/or mood-altering drugs, including Valium, Prozac, or Xanax which, besides being addictive, further aggravate the problem by suppressing the real cause. These drugs worsen the condition by deepening the depression, both physical and mental. Once patients become dependent upon these agents, brain chemistry becomes altered. Then, it may take weeks or months to normalize brain chemical levels. Anti-depressants and anti-anxiety medications cause a unique disease, Neurotransmitter Depletion Syndrome, another syndrome to add to the list.

Here is an important point: the brain contains its own natural antidepressants. It has been found that medicines which numb the brain, Valium, Xanax, Zoloft, Prozac, narcotics, codeine, and the like wreak havoc with the natural chemicals that control mood. These chemicals, known as *neurotransmitters*, include such compounds as tryptophan, serotonin, norepinephrine, acetylcholine, gamma-amino butyric acid, and epinephrine. The fact is such drugs cause potentially permanent damage of the neurochemical system.

There is another category of brain chemicals: the *endorphins*. These are the brain's natural painkillers. Endorphin levels are also depressed by medications. Refined sugar also depletes them.

It is of utmost importance to reduce or eliminate all mood-altering drugs in order to cure migraines. A list of medications which inhibit the function and/or synthesis of neurotransmitters/endorphins includes:

- barbiturates
- Demerol
- Dilantin
- Tylenol #3
- Xanax
- Dalmane
- Zoloft
- morphine
- Halcion
- Restoril
- Valium
- codeine
- Prozac
- Paxil

In contrast, thyroid hormones help speed up the synthesis of these important natural brain chemicals. Depression is not a sign of a drug deficiency. It is a signal that natural chemicals are deficient, including thyroxine (thyroid hormone). Giving thyroid extract is a natural way to curb depression, as well as other mood disorders, without the side effects that commonly result from taking mood-altering medications.

The Thyroid and the Immune System

The health of the immune system is closely tied to how well the thyroid gland is functioning. From reading this book it should become clear that healthy immunity is one of the best preventatives against migraines. This is because the immune cells and their secretions act as guardians, protecting the body from the harmful chemical reactions that occur as a result of food or chemical allergies. Untold billions of immune cells line the digestive tract, lymph tissues, and blood vessels. They lie in wait for allergens and/or microbes, so they can detoxify and destroy them. In addition, immune organs, such as the spleen, liver, lymph nodes, and thymus, contain innumerable amounts of these cells.

Hypothyroid individuals exhibit impaired immunity. This is largely a consequence of the role the thyroid gland in controlling body temperature. Hypothyroid patients exhibit a significant measurable reduction in body temperature. Sometimes the chill of hypothyroidism goes all the way to the bone. This can be a major problem. It is within the bone, specifically the bone marrow, that most immune cells are made. Proper synthesis of these cells is dependent upon a normal body temperature. Even a slightly high temperature is better than a low temperature. This is what happens with a fever. A natural stimulant, fever provokes the bone marrow and immune organs to synthesize white blood cells to destroy the toxin or invader. In contrast, even a slight drop in body temperature leads to reduced synthesis of white cells, often by the billions. The lower the temperature becomes, the greater the impairment is in cell synthesis. Therefore, the end result for the migraine patient is that fewer white cells are available to combat allergic reactions as well as infection. As a result, the migraines will be more frequent, prolonged, and severe. An improvement in thyroid function helps maximize the immune response, and this may aid in eliminating the headaches permanently.

The thyroid gland is highly sensitive to stress. Prolonged emotional stress may cause significant thyroid impairment. In fact, stress can burn out the thyroid quicker than anything else. People who are long term sugar addicts usually have thyroid problems, since this substance causes thyroid burnout. Other substances which impair thyroid function include pesticides, herbicides, dioxins, solvents, hydrocarbons, heavy metals, fluoride, and chlorine. Heavy metals, such as lead, cadmium, mercury, and aluminum, bind to the enzymes needed to synthesize thyroid hormones. This is also the mechanism by which fluoride and chlorine exert their toxic effects. People who drink fluoridated water, use fluoride toothpaste, or take fluoride rinses are at risk for thyroid damage. Fluoride is one of the most destructive substances known against the thyroid.

In extreme cases hypothyroidism can prove debilitating or even life-threatening. Only a small minority develop the disease to this degree. More commonly, chronic low-level illness results. A list of diseases associated with thyroid failure includes:

- chronic candidiasis
- Epstein-Barr syndrome
- coronary artery disease
- high blood pressure
- lupus
- obesity
- migraine headaches
- atherosclerosis
  (hardening of the arteries)

- diabetes
- osteoarthritis
- hypoglycemia
- intestinal parasites
- rheumatoid arthritis
- Raynaud's Disease
- eczema
- psoriasis

Not every person with migraines has hypothyroidism. However, regarding those with daily or weekly migraines the likelihood for a thyroid abnormality is high. Such individuals would surely respond by the daily intake of ThyroAid as well as the potent anti-inflammatory herbal extract, Migraten. In these cases it is extremely likely that through correction of the thyroid impairment significant improvement in the headaches will result. This can be done through prescriptions, but in many cases it is sufficient to take the ThyroAid as well as change the diet, eliminating all refined sugar, processed foods, and food additives. Eliminating the intake of chlorinated water would also be helpful. What's more, Migraten can be taken on a daily basis as a preventive. As a result, overall health will be enhanced, allergies will be minimized, and depression plus fatigue will largely be eliminated. These positive, comprehensive results are only to be expected by improving the function of a gland known as the Master of Metabolism.

Adrenal Insufficiency

While the thyroid gland is the master of metabolism, it is the adrenal glands that are truly the masters of all hormone glands. By themselves the adrenal glands out-produce all other endocrine glands combined in terms of total numbers of hormones. Over 45 hormones are synthesized in these small glands which are somewhat smaller than golf balls. The adrenals are found atop each kidney.

Anatomically, these glands can be divided into two sectors. These are the *adrenal cortex* and the *adrenal medulla*. The medulla is the inside or center of the gland. Its primary function is to synthesize *adrenaline* and *noradrenaline*. These hormones are responsible for numerous functions. Most notable is the so-called "fight or flight" reaction. Have you ever become so startled that you became "scared stiff"? Or, have you ever gotten into a heated argument to the point where you were "ready to fight"? Both of these responses are mediated by a surge of adrenaline. On the other hand have you ever become so scared that you got a sudden burst of energy to "run like crazy," as would happen to a person being chased by a ferocious dog? This, of course, is the flight response.

Adrenaline is the agent which helps athletes become mentally prepared or "psyched up" for their competitive events. It is the chemical which flows through the blood when we are frightened by a loud noise or when we experience the fear of impending doom. Adrenaline prepares the human body for all manner of daily activities, plus some risky and unusual ones as well.

Most adrenal hormones are synthesized in the cortex which is the outer part of the gland. Cortisol, or natural cortisone, is the most dominant of these. After being produced, some hormones are stored, while a certain fixed amount is secreted directly into the bloodstream. Cortisol levels are greatest in the morning between 7:00 and 8:30. In a sense, cortical is the body's wake-up chemical.

Cortical hormones have a wide range of functions and exert significant control over the operation of the digestive, immune and nervous systems. There is hardly a single function of the human body that is not influenced by these hormones. Some of the functions/effects of adrenal steroids, particularly cortical, include:

1) the maintenance of normal blood sugar levels

2) increased metabolism or breakdown of protein

3) increased breakdown of fats, and in some cases increased deposition of fats

4) suppression of white blood cell synthesis

5) suppression of immune or allergic responses

6) irritability of the nervous system

7) increased production of stomach acid

8) increased bladder pressure and urination

9) increased loss of sodium, potassium, and water through the urine

People who are under stress secrete excess amounts of cortisol. It takes little imagination to comprehend the potential problems resulting from over-secretion. Excess cortisone, whether natural or synthetic, leads to suppression of the immune system to the degree that harm can be done to the internal organs. Affected organs include the stomach, intestines, liver, pancreas, spleen, thymus, and kidneys.

The concept that thousands of Americans have malfunctioning, over-stressed adrenal glands was first introduced in the early 1940s by a brilliant endocrinologist, John Tintera, M.D. The validity of Dr. Tintera's work was supported and confirmed by the internationally renowned researcher, Hans Selye, who spent much of his life studying the negative effects of stress upon animals and humans.

Dr. Tintera's major findings included the determination that many of his patients suffered from a syndrome of impaired adrenal function, a condition he called *sub-clinical Addison's Disease*. In coining this syndrome Dr. Tintera went against the established medical views of his time. As with many originators he was ostracized. Yet, his work survived in a book called *"Hypoadrenocorticism"* published by the Adrenal Metabolic Research Society. Dr. Tintera's original research and observations can be found in this book.

Tintera believed that the standard medical view of adrenal disorders was incomplete. The medical profession holds that the adrenal glands are involved in disease only when frank symptoms of total adrenal failure—Addison's Disease—or when symptoms of the adrenal excess—Cushing's Syndrome—exist. No doubt, both these diseases are serious and are often life-threatening. However, there must be an in-between. Must a person always have a serious disease before a diagnosis can be made? According to Dr. Tintera there is an intermediate symptom, and millions of Americans have it.

If the reader has chronic, severe migraines, especially the types which are resistant to pain medicines, it is likely that adrenal dysfunction exists. This disorder is known medically as *adrenal insufficiency* or *hypoadrenocorticism*. Both terms indicate that the adrenal glands either are no longer producing the right balance of hormones, or they are unable to produce enough cortical hormones. In other words, the adrenal glands are functioning in an insufficient fashion in respect to the number of stresses that exist in life. Pain is a stress, and the weakened adrenals are unable to cope with the elements which provoke headache pain. By strengthening the adrenal glands, the resistance against migraines would greatly improve.

How did the adrenal glands get in such bad shape? What could possibly have made them so weak? Why do weak adrenals cause individuals to be susceptible to pain and migraines, and why do they make a person vulnerable to allergic reactions? These questions will be answered in the following sections.

Refined Carbohydrates — An Adrenal Poison?

The adrenal glands can be readily disrupted. They can be greatly affected by poor diet. These glands are involved in the metabolism of sugars, starches, fats, and proteins; in other words, food. The role played by the adrenals in fat and protein metabolism is relatively minor in comparison to that played in carbohydrate metabolism. Carbohydrates are sugars and starches.

It is the refined carbohydrates which greatly stress these adrenal glands. The worst of these are the refined sugars—white sugar, corn syrup, maple syrup, molasses, fructose, glucose, dextrose, and malt. White flour and white rice are less stress-causing, but not by much. Refined sugars and starches are devitalized, nutritionally deficient foods. All they do is pack a calorie load—a sugar fix, if you will. These foods place great stress on the adrenal glands, increasing the demand for the synthesis of adrenal hormones. Little, short of severe emotional stress, can weaken the adrenals more significantly than a load of refined carbohydrates.

For most Americans refined carbohydrates form a major part of the diet. The average consumption of sugar in the United

States is a whopping 150 pounds per person per year. Each year this amount rises. Thus, correspondingly, the incidence of adrenal insufficiency is rising.

Some people claim that they don't eat much sugar. It is true that certain nutritionally aware people have dramatically curbed their sugar intake. However, most Americans consume excessive amounts, and if they don't currently, they probably did at one time.

Think back a little. Did you eat loads of junk food as a child, teenager, or adult? Go all the way back. Was your mother a sugar/starch addict, eating such things as ice cream, candy, cookies, pastries, pop, white bread, or white rice, while you were still in the womb? As an infant were you nursed on corn syrup-laced formulas, or were you given sugar water in or out of the hospital? Were you fed sugar-infested cereals for breakfast as a toddler? Or, did you receive fist-loads of sugar as a small child in the form of grandma's goodies, candies, lollipops, jawbreakers, jelly beans, cookies, candy bars, doughnuts, ice cream, shakes, malts, pastries, pop-tarts, birthday cakes, caramels, taffy, and gum? Did you guzzle Kool-Aid, Tang, Ovaltine, Nestle's Quik, Hershey's Chocolate Syrup in milk, chocolate milk, Hi-C, orangeade, lemonade, fruit punch, or similar sugar-loaded drinks? As a toddler or teenager did you drink loads of soda pop each day or every week? Were desserts of homemade or store-bought bakery goods, pies, doughnuts, and cakes on the daily or weekly menu? Did you junk out on sugar whenever and wherever you could?

Was white bread, white flour, or pasta a staple at your home? Were crackers such as saltines, Ritz, Waverly Wafers, Wheat Thins, Cheez Nips, and graham crackers common snack items? How often did you consume a bunch of cookies, whether homemade or store bought—Oreos, Hydrox, butter, oatmeal, Ginger Snaps, chocolate chip, Pinwheels, peanut butter, Pepperidge Farms, Snack Ways, or Archway? Did you often indulge in Twinkies, cupcakes, Snow Balls, Suzie-Qs, Ding Dongs, fruit pies, or Little Debbies? What about candy bars— Mars bars, Three Muskateers, Snickers, KitKats, O'Henrys, Butterfingers, Baby Ruths, Hersheys, Nestles, M&Ms, Reese's Peanut Butter Cups, Mounds, Almond Joys and similar sugar-loaded aggressors? Did you continuously bombard your gut with these or similar adrenal bombs? Most likely you did. There are very few exceptions, at least for anyone born since the late 1930s. The rule is if a person lived in the USA during the 1940s through the 1990s and is under 70 years old, he/she ate enormous amounts of sugar in the form of sugar and flour-infested gut bombs, or in the form of sugar "blended into the food supply." As a result, most Americans have probably destroyed their adrenal function. In addition to the gut bombs, sugar entered the diet in more disguised forms, that is foods to which sugar is added. Cole slaw, ketchup, tartar sauce, salad dressings, bologna, hot dogs, corned beef, pork'n beans, relish, spaghetti sauce, barbecue sauce, canned herring, and canned corn are just a few examples.

Are there exceptions—are there people who have lived a "sugar-free" life? They would be people who had the fortune of having highly educated, nutritionally oriented mothers and grandmothers who kept virtually all sources of refined sugar out of the house, and who monitored the diet of the children while they were at school or play. Do you know anyone who fits this description? There is another exception. It would be those individuals who naturally have huge powerful adrenal glands, which are able to withstand this sugar-induced adrenal stress.

If you don't fit one of these categories, then you must avoid all dangerous processed foods if you wish to remain healthy, energetic, and free of migraines. This is a rule that can't be broken, if success is to come quickly in curing the headaches.

Synthetic chemicals cause adrenal stress. Various fumes may agitate these glands. Alcohol also significantly stresses them. This is particularly true in the quantities in which it is consumed by alcoholics. Invariably, alcoholics have weak adrenals. They crave alcohol in order to get a lift. Smokers use cigarettes for an adrenal boost. The same is true of drug addicts. This is one reason drinkers continue drinking, smokers continue smoking, and drug addicts continue their addiction. Such addicts are continually prodding their adrenals to gain a temporary high. Nicotine gives smokers an adrenaline kick. However, this artificial stimulation ultimately results in a state of dire adrenal exhaustion. This is why they must continually "light up another."

Stress and the Adrenal Glands

In many illnesses emotional and psychic stresses are the major causes of adrenal failure, playing even more of a role than diet. This kind of stress can lead to everything from weak adrenals to heart disease, heart attacks, stroke, arthritis, colitis, ulcers, and cancer. Here are just a few examples of how mental stress can lead to physical damage:

1. Stress causes platelet levels in the blood to increase and also causes platelets to become more sticky. Because of this, blood clots may form more easily. Migraines are associated with an increased degree of platelet adhesiveness.

2. Medical students undertaking exams exhibit a measurable decline in immune function, which increases their susceptibility to colds and flu.

3. Hans Selye found that anger causes a massive increase in the secretion of stomach acid and that this excess acid damages the intestinal walls. He also found that anger, excitement, and/or worry significantly stress the adrenal glands, increasing the secretion of adrenal hormones.

4. Researchers known as neuroendocrinologists have found that stress causes the production of certain chemicals called neurohormones. These chemicals are very powerful and can initiate the degenerative changes that lead to many diseases, including cancer, heart disease, and arthritis.

Mental stress can cause illness or it can worsen existing illnesses. To understand how adrenal stress contributes to migraines the work of Tintera must be reviewed. It was stated previously that two of the major causes of migraines are allergies and low blood sugar. Adrenal insufficiency contributes to both of these. As stated by Dr. Tintera, "The chief complaints listed for patients with hypoadrenocorticism are often similar to those found in persons who are hypoglycemic." What were these suspect symptoms? They included weakness, fatigue, mood swings, headaches, and faintness. Dr. Tintera found these symptoms were, in fact, due to fluctuations in blood sugar levels and the severity of the symptoms correlated with the lowest sugar readings. He also found that any sudden emotional upset led to further drops in blood sugar levels. Thus, when blood sugar levels were low, patients were more likely to be depressed, anxious, and psychotic. Dr. Tintera quoted the work of another researcher, who reported that when experiencing emotional stress, business executives had definite drops in blood sugar levels.

The above data confirms that the mind affects the body. In fact, it largely controls it. Regarding migraine these sudden drops in blood sugar levels are a major factor. When this happens, great stress is placed on all organs, particularly the brain. The brain uses 80% of the glucose consumed by the body. A sudden migraine attack is often the end result of this stress. When a rapid decline in blood sugar occurs, the body attempts to rectify the problem by raising blood sugar levels to normal. This is where the adrenal glands play a critical role.

Healthy adrenal glands "kick in" by secreting the appropriate hormones to bring blood sugar levels back to normal. The weaker the adrenals are, the longer it takes for this mechanism to come into play. The result may be a prolonged battle with severe hypoglycemic migraine.

Some people believe that the answer to this type of headache is a sugar fix. It is true that eating foods high in sugar might raise blood sugar levels, but this rise would be temporary. The added stress caused by the refined sugar would further disrupt adrenal function, making it that much more difficult for these glands to stabilize blood sugar levels.

Raw honey is a possible exception to this rule. Some headaches may actually be relieved by the consumption of large quantities of pure, unadulterated honey. What is pure honey? It is honey which has undergone minimal or no processing. Basically, this means the honey is extracted directly from the hive without undergoing excessive heating or straining. However, the honey need not be fresh, since its potency remains intact over time. Honey was found in Egyptian tombs, and it still was edible. A special note: crude raw honey is defined as honey in which the bees are never fed sugar. In the United States such honeys are rare. To order truly non-sugar fed bee honey, which is 100% wild and raw, call 1-800-243-5242.

Patients may respond to consuming three to four ounces of pure honey several times during the day. A word of caution: honey only works for headaches due to fluctuations in blood sugar levels. Also, diabetics and severe hypoglycemics must avoid honey or any other simple sugar.

Allergy itself is a form of adrenal stress, since these glands are largely responsible for the anti-allergy coping mechanism. The connection is clear; adrenal insufficiency allows allergic reactions to proceed to an excess, which leads to headaches. The severity and number of allergies is directly related to the degree of adrenal weakness. People with chronic adrenal fatigue tend to have 30 to 50 food allergies.

A classic example of adrenal-induced allergy is the perfume/fume sensitivity syndrome. People who experience this are reactive to virtually any artificial and also many natural odors. Invariably, fatigued adrenals are the cause. This hypoadrenal state leads to a heightened smell sensitivity which is, incredibly, some 100,000 times the normal. When the underlying adrenal disorder is treated, this chemical odor sensitivity is improved, and the allergic migraines caused by fumes or other synthetic substances will dissipate. It should also be noted that the symptoms of adrenal failure and allergy are similar. Chemical and food-sensitive individuals nearly always fit the picture of the hypoadrenal condition. The more severe the sensitivity, the weaker are the adrenals.

So many symptoms result from adrenal problems that it would be difficult to mention them all. A list of the more common ones is provided as a simple test. Take this test to determine the existence of adrenal problems and to also determine the severity:

Adrenal Insufficiency Exam

	Yes	No
Do You Experience:		
1. constant fatigue	☐	☐
2. nervousness	☐	☐
3. irritability	☐	☐
4. depression	☐	☐
5. episodes of weakness	☐	☐

6. lightheadedness ☐ ☐

7. fainting spells ☐ ☐

8. headaches ☐ ☐

9. heart palpitations ☐ ☐

10. cravings for salt ☐ ☐

11. cravings for sweets ☐ ☐

12. intolerance to alcohol ☐ ☐

13. intolerance to cigarette smoke ☐ ☐

14. alternating diarrhea and constipation ☐ ☐

15. hard, pebble-like stools ☐ ☐

16. vague heartburn or indigestion ☐ ☐

17. vague pains or digestive discomfort in the
abdomen ☐ ☐

18. food reactions/allergies ☐ ☐

19. lack of appetite ☐ ☐

20. premenstrual symptom ☐ ☐

21. pains in the lower neck and upper back ☐ ☐

22. pain or tightness in the upper neck or scalp ☐ ☐

23. inability to concentrate ☐ ☐

24. fears and anxiety ☐ ☐

25. periods of confusion ☐ ☐

26. impaired memory ☐ ☐

27. frustration ☐ ☐

28. compulsive behavior ☐ ☐

29. tendency towards heat exhaustion ☐ ☐

30. cold hands and feet ☐ ☐

31. clammy, sweaty hands and/or feet ☐ ☐

32. a sense of well being after eating, especially
the evening meal ☐ ☐

33. difficulty relaxing (unless working) ☐ ☐

34. excessive sweating of the palms and feet ☐ ☐

35. depression relieved by eating ☐ ☐

36. heartburn aggravated by stress ☐ ☐

37. night urination (after falling asleep) ☐ ☐

38. a tendency to have guilt feelings ☐ ☐

39. extreme sensitivity to smells ☐ ☐

40. extreme sensitivity to noises ☐ ☐

41. inability to cope with stressful events ☐ ☐

42. tendency to cry easily ☐ ☐

_____

SCORE
(calculated by the number of questions answered yes)

1-9   This score indicates that adrenal insufficiency is likely but is probably not necessarily the primary cause of health problems. Even so, the treatment of even minimal adrenal dysfunction will result in improved health, and headaches may be diminished.

10-20   Adrenal insufficiency is probably a major cause of health problems. To treat this a special diet low in refined sugars and starches is advised (See Dr. Ingram's book, *How to Eat Right and Live Longer*). In addition, if the underlying adrenal disorder is resolved through nutritional and hormonal treatment, the migraine tendency will be greatly improved. Here, AdrenoAid, four capsules every morning, is invaluable. Treatment also includes the use of adrenal-enhancing nutrients such as pantothenic acid, thiamine, vitamin C, vitamin A, vitamin E, vitamin B-6, Coenzyme Q-10, and carnitine.

21-29   This score indicates the existence of severe adrenal insufficiency. Such individuals usually have a history of sugar or starch addiction. A history of alcoholism and/or smoking may also be found. Treatment consists of radical changes in diet, vitamin-mineral supplementation, the addition of crude royal jelly, that is AdrenoAid, six capsules every morning, and adrenal-enhancing herbs such as ginseng, garlic, and licorice root. Take also Royal Oil, 1 teaspoon daily as well as the aforementioned adrenal-enhancing nutrients.

30-42   The diagnosis of subclinical adrenal failure applies. Medical diagnosis and treatment is advised. Treatment should be immediate in order to prevent the condition from worsening. Measures such as those mentioned above should be instituted, and special medications may be required. These must be prescribed under a doctor's care. They include thyroid hormone, natural cortisone, intravenous B-5 and B-6, and intravenous minerals such as magnesium and calcium. Take also the aforementioned adrenal-boosting nutrients. A more natural approach is to take crude fortified royal jelly, that is the AdrenoAid. This formula readily regulates the adrenals. Take six capsules every morning with breakfast and another two at noon. Also, take Royal Oil under the tongue, 1 teaspoon twice daily. Many individuals will improve dramatically once the diet is changed and appropriate nutritional supplementation is prescribed.

Patients with adrenal insufficiency are unable to respond positively to combat the toxicity of allergic reactions. Thus, eating the allergenic food leads to symptoms. Until the immune system and adrenal glands become strong enough to cope with the allergies, symptoms will persist. Therefore, it is crucial to utilize a curative approach to rebuild and repair these organs. This is so the allergic individual can cope with life and live a reasonably normal existence on this earth. The American public is looking for safer, less invasive treatments. The medical profession must step up to the challenge and provide these alternative, nontoxic treatments.

To understand the logic behind chronic illness all that is necessary is to evaluate the underlying physiology. Just by understanding the mechanisms of the function of the human body, things begin to make sense. Always remember the old adage coined by the father of Osteopathic Medicine, Dr. Andrew Taylor Still, who said, "Find it, fix it, then leave it be." This powerful statement summarizes the entire philosophy of osteopathy. This philosophy can be applied to migraines and virtually all other diseases.

Chapter 6

Structural Therapies

Manipulation: A Science or an Art?

Osteopathic or chiropractic manipulative treatment (OMT/CMT) could prove to be a boon to the migraine patient. Manipulative treatment has been used for centuries as an adjunct in the treatment of illness. While there is a certain degree of science to it, OMT/CMT is primarily an art. It is a skill of the hands, of touch, of manual dexterity, and of technique. It involves precision, quickness, and agility. These are hardly the skills of a scientist.

It is important to understand that the quality of OMT/CMT is directly related to the skill of the operator. The strength of the operator is not nearly as important as his/her technique. In fact, brute strength may be more of an impediment than an asset. The old adage, "The rougher the treatment, the better it feels", has no place in the art of skillful manipulative treatment.

This chapter will serve as a guide to the selection of a skillful manipulative therapist. There are hundreds of excellent OMT/CMT specialists throughout the country. Some of these physicians specialize in areas such as *cranial-sacral treatment*, sports medicine, low back pain, occupational injuries, etc.

While few specialize in headache treatment per se, most have on record case after case of patients whose headaches improved or disappeared following manipulative treatments.

There are a few steps to take before undergoing this type of therapy. First, do some checking about the skills and reputation of the doctor before making any decision. Determine what type of technique he/she uses. Avoid "neck poppers," that is, practitioners who treat migraines by simply manipulating the neck only. Spinal manipulation is often contraindicated *during acute migraine crisis.* In most instances it is unwise to manipulate the neck during or at the onset of a migraine. Often, this serves only to aggravate the headache. It is preferable to wait until the headache is gone and then correct any neck lesions.

Many doctors manipulate the neck during migraine attacks with good intentions and the patient's blessings. This is understandable—the pain is so agonizing that both the doctor and patient wish to attempt anything that could possibly bring relief. Yet, the severe, throbbing type of migraine rarely responds to this type of manipulative treatment, that is during the migraine crisis. Some patients find more gentle techniques such as muscle energy, soft tissue, pressure point, and cranial sacral therapy to be an exception to this rule. Yet, in contrast dull low-grade tension headaches frequently can be relieved by the use of manipulative techniques, and this relief is often immediate.

There is another rule. Any time manipulative treatment causes pain, avoid it. In this instance the definition of pain is any discomfort that lasts for days or weeks after a treatment. If necessary, seek a different practitioner who uses a more gentle technique. If pain is created as a result of the manipulative treatment, it should be mild and should disappear within 72 hours. This might be a normal result of being "realigned." This means that the muscles become sore due to assuming new postures, and the soreness should disappear within a few days. However, pain which persists despite the lapse of adequate time is abnormal. Receiving further treatments would be inadvisable.

Few therapies have the attribute of being free of side effects. Surgery has numerous side effects, and so does anesthesia. Medications can cause tissue damage, much of it permanent. Even certain vitamins can be toxic if taken in high enough doses. Some people have died from drinking too much water.

To be afraid may prove self-destructive, but to proceed with caution is wise. Regarding your health, be careful before making sudden decisions. Make sure you feel comfortable with your doctor; this instinctual response is equally as important as any investigation that might be performed. Avoid doing things just to please the doctor. Try instead to please yourself.

Manipulative medicine can be good medicine. It was one of Andrew Taylor Still's favorite remedies. He specified osteopathic manipulation. There are also many good chiropractors. Manipulation has helped thousands, with ailments ranging from arthritis to aching feet. A partial list of the conditions which may respond to skillful manipulative treatment include:

• arthritis	• asthma
• backache	• breathing disorders
• bronchitis	• bursitis
• chronic fatigue	• headache
• hip pain	• knee pain
• neck sprain or whiplash	• pinched nerve
• sacroiliac strain	• sciatica
• scoliosis	• shoulder pain
• upper back pain	

Tension headache is the type that best responds to OMT/CMT. Often, the response is so beneficial that no other treatment is required. With migraines it is usually a different story. OMT/CMT acts more as an adjunctive therapy than an outright cure. However, when combined with trigger point treatment, allergy removal, and hormonal support it offers significant benefits.

Why OMT/CMT Works

Manipulation directly affects the structural components of the body. The goal is to improve the mechanical function of the joints. However, there is an additional benefit of improved structure and body mechanics. The functions of the body chemistry and internal organs also improve. Structure does affect functional operations: how we breathe, how we metabolize, how we synthesize, how we circulate, and how we eliminate.

Balanced structure also means greater energy. This can be explained by the laws of body mechanics. It takes a greater amount of energy to operate a body which has spinal lesions and joint strains than one which is free of them. This can be best visualized by comparing the human body to a machine. If a bearing is grinding or is stuck, it takes enormous energy to drive the machine. The machine can actually burn out its motor due to the strain. If the bearing is repaired, the mechanism runs smoothly again and much less energy is required. A similar process occurs in the human body when a joint is "stuck." The negative effects are not as dramatic as would be seen in a solid metal machine, because the body is flexible and can compensate. However, the loss of energy does happen, and chronic fatigue may result. If the lesion is in the right spot, there may also be headaches. If various joint strains are normalized, invariably, the person will feel better, and, often, the incidence of headaches will be reduced.

Numerous structural disorders of the spine may have a negative bearing on human health and body mechanics. Many of these either cause headaches or serve to increase headache frequency and/or severity. In true fashion the tailbone is connected to the hip bone, and the hip bone to the back bone, and the back bone to the neck. Just because headaches start in the head and neck, it doesn't mean this is where the major problem lies. The primary lesion might be elsewhere such as the tailbone or lower back. These regions will now be segregated for further explanation.

Neck Injuries

Regarding migraines, injuries to the delicate structures of the neck tend to aggravate the condition. Car accidents are a common cause of neck injuries. Millions suffer with chronic pain as a result of whiplash-type injuries. Whiplash is known technically as *acceleration/deceleration injury*. It is so named because the neck follows the path of the impact in rear end collisions. The neck is first jammed forward, then backward, and then forward again. Tremendous forces come into play, even in low speed impacts. These types of injury are extremely traumatic, and a great deal of effort is often required to normalize the tissues. The neck is highly flexible and mobile; it simply gives way and is severely twisted, strained and torqued. Frequently, the neck becomes so weak as a result of stretching of the muscles that it fatigues under the weight of the head. These symptoms may be descriptively called the Whiplash Triad: fatigue of the muscles, neck and jaw pain as well as headache—a combination which is often difficult to cure.

Other neck trauma may result from falls or athletic injuries. The common "pinched nerve" of the neck responds exceedingly well to manipulative treatment. Thus, headaches caused by pinched nerves are usually easily abated.

The Anatomy of the Neck

The neck can be divided into two sections: the upper part and the lower part. Strain upon the upper neck is of particular importance, since this is where the first three cervical nerves arise—C 1, C2, and C3. These nerves carry the sensory fibers which are responsible for pain in the headache regions of the scalp—the posterior scalp or occiput, the temples and the frontal-sinus area. The nerves originate within the upper reaches of the spinal cord from which they exit through small canals in the second, third, and fourth cervical vertebrae. Even slight strain upon the vertebrae, muscles, or ligaments of this region can result in pain or make the nerves hyper-irritable. Therefore, as a result of such a strain, the risk for headaches increases.

The best way to relax impinged or hypersensitive nerves is to utilize structural treatment aimed at releasing the strain. It could be massage, acupuncture, trigger point therapy, manipulation, or physical therapy. However, manipulative treatment is often the quickest and easiest way to achieve results. Medications are usually ineffective, since nerve impingement is a mechanical problem, not a chemical one. Mechanical treatment, and manipulation usually work wonders—and, at times, miracles.

Mid to Upper Back

The upper and middle portion of the back have an interesting connection with headaches. This region is the site where special nerves, called *sympathetic fibers,* arise. Like the cervical nerves, these nerves originate within the spinal cord and exit through small canals in the vertebrae. Some of the sympathetic nerves travel directly upward into the neck and head. Others travel directly to the internal organs.

In respect to headaches what is the importance of the sympathetic nerves? They are the prime nerve system for controlling blood flow within the brain. Blood is the primary conduit for the delivery of nourishment, including oxygen. Oxygen is crucial to life. A lack of it disturbs body chemistry. Pain and inflammation usually result. For its weight the brain uses a greater amount of oxygen than any other organ. It is ultra sensitive to oxygen deprivation. Excessive discharge from the sympathetic nerves can diminish oxygen supplies to the brain by reducing blood flow. This is because overstimulation of these nerves causes cranial blood vessels to constrict, which reduces oxygen delivery to the cells. When pain-sensitive structures of the cranium are deprived of oxygen, extreme pain results. Many who have had heart or neck artery surgery are familiar with how severe this kind of pain can be. During these procedures blood flow to the brain is actually cut off, which results in severe oxygen deprivation. To watch one of these patients writhe in pain is a vivid reminder of how sensitive the brain is to reduced oxygen supply.

Researchers have proven that structural imbalance and/or trauma of the upper thoracic spine may alter the function of the sympathetics. Here again manipulative treatment can prove invaluable and is usually the most effective method for reversing structural defects.

Peripheral nerves of the head and neck are also involved in migraines. These nerves are responsible for the sensation of pain in superficial tissues, including the skin and the layers just under the skin.

A number of trigger points are found in the thoracic spine. When pressed, many of these will radiate a sensation directly upward toward the neck and/or scalp. For headache sufferers it is particularly important to eliminate these triggers. The triggers are often concentrated along the middle of the spine, or they may be found in significant numbers about the shoulder blade. Some headache triggers are found in such distant sites as the hands and arms. In fact, there is an important acupuncture headache point in the outer part of the hand, just up from the base of the little finger. Another one exists between the thumb and the forefinger.

The complexity of the human nervous system never ceases to amaze and confound both scientists and scholars. Science has been able to comprehend only a crude, simplistic understanding of it. Even so, what is essential is what works clinically, not so much how it works. Structural therapy, including manipulation, trigger point injections, and acupuncture, can eradicate many of these triggers with a resultant reduction in headache pain.

The Lower Back

Lower back problems may cause or aggravate headaches. This may not come as much of a surprise. It is common for patients to say that they get a headache when their "back is out." However, few people understand the mechanism. The lower back is vulnerable to strain and injury more so than any other region of the spine. Low back strain/sprain is one of the most common ailments occurring in America today. There are many different types of low back conditions, including slipped disc, lumbar sprain, lumbago, pinched nerve, subluxation, sciatica, sacroiliac sprain, or the more severe ruptured disc.

Whenever there is a lower back injury of any sort, it must be remembered that the lower back has a direct connection to the upper neck and the base of the skull. This connection is via a special membrane known as the *dura*. The dura is the protective membrane which encases the spinal cord. As the spinal cord ends in the lower regions of the back, so does the dura. The dura is anchored in the lower back to a region just a few inches below the lowest lumbar vertebra (L5) on a bone known as the *sacrum*. In the neck it is tightly fixed to the 2nd and 3rd cervical vertebra. In the skull it has numerous attachments, which include the occiput and all cranial bones. The occiput is the large bone in the back where the neck meets the skull.

The key concept is that the dura is inelastic. It does not give, not even a fraction of an inch. Ligaments and muscles also connect the neck and skull to the lower back. However, there is a certain amount of give to these. Not so with the dura. If it is put under strain, it will pull on all its attachments. Now the importance of these interconnections becomes clear. Strain on the lower back puts pressure on the lower attachments of the dura, which pulls on the neck and head. This causes nerve tension and/or impingement, and the end result is pain.

The Tailbone

A discussion of the mechanical causes of head pain would be incomplete without including the tailbone. The tailbone is known anatomically as the *coccyx*. The dura attaches firmly here, covering most of it. Many people with chronic headaches have a history of a severe fall on the rump, such as slipping on ice, or a fall from a height, etc. In such instances it is possible that the headaches are partly due to a broken or dislocated tailbone. These individuals may find it difficult to sit on a hard surface and will be forced to favor one side for comfort. The person who squirms when sitting on a hard surface surely has a damaged tailbone. Other common complaints resulting from tailbone injuries include leg cramps, leg pain, difficulty taking long strides, bladder pressure, one-sided leg swelling, ankle pain, and constipation.

The tailbone can be realigned through manipulative therapy. However, severe trauma can result in permanent damage. In this case surgical correction may be necessary.

In summary, structural problems often lead to functional disturbances. This is the primary basis of the osteopathic philosophy. It should not come as a surprise that migraines or other headaches can result from structural defects. Until the mechanical/structural imbalances are corrected, it is likely that the susceptibility to pain will remain. Appropriate treatment may include quality care from an osteopathic physician, chiropractor, or from a medical physician skilled in structural or manipulative treatment.

Trigger Point Injections

Nothing, short of avoiding allergic foods, has so dramatic an effect on headaches as trigger point injections. These unique injections can help relieve and/or cure migraines. They are invaluable for treating headaches caused by muscular tension. This technique is also invaluable for *TMJ*-related headaches. The fact is point injections are useful in virtually any type of headache not due to serious underlying disease.

The term "trigger point" is certainly a graphic one. That's because points of pain exist along headache regions in the scalp, temples, and base of the head/neck. Many headache patients are familiar with these triggers. Often, pressing on them provides relief, although it is usually temporary. However, a true trigger is one which, when pressed, conducts a nerve sensation—a tingle of sorts—to another region. Usually, the trigger sends its impulse in a linear fashion, either up or down, from the point pressed. One need not press hard, since most triggers are found just under the skin. For example, a person experiencing a headache located primarily over the eye or behind the eye will often experience a shooting trigger reaction when certain occipital points are pressed. For headaches localized on the side of the head (the temple), triggers are usually found along the same side of the neck and in the scalp over the temporal region. In headaches localized to the back of the neck triggers are almost exclusively found there in both the neck and scalp. In fact, in most types of headaches trigger points are found in the posterior scalp and neck.

The exact nature of trigger points—what they consist of and what causes them—is unknown. Could trigger points act surreptitiously as guides for the practitioner to uncover the origin of the pain? It is sufficient to presume that they are sites of concentrated pain stimuli. This is the closest definition that can be found.

Most experts agree that, while many structures deep within the skull are sensitive to pain, headache pain arises primarily from structures outside the skull. This fact is apparent to any headache sufferer who well knows how painful the scalp, eye sockets, forehead, and neck become during a headache. Pain can originate from inside the skull (*intracranially*), and, often, it feels as if this is where much of the pain arises from. Yet, researchers have found that headaches are usually caused by inflammation and irritation of pain sensitive structures such as nerves, arteries, muscle fibers, tendons, and fascia located *extracranially*. Although it feels like the pain is all in the head, it is usually mostly outside the head.

The intracranial arteries, nerves, and veins are sensitive to pain. However, in terms of treatment the pain that is important is that which occurs in the superficial tissues. Most of this pain is concentrated just under the skin of the scalp, face, and neck. These are the regions where most trigger points are found.

Trigger points also exist at sites seemingly unrelated to the pain such as the hands, feet, shoulders, upper back, and lower back. Often, when these triggers are touched, pain radiates directly to the headache region. In some cases it is just as important to treat these distant triggers as it is to correct the local ones.

Trauma is one of the most common causes of trigger points. In addition, many chronic illnesses are associated with their development. Bowel disorders, including constipation and colitis, are highly correlated. Arthritics, especially rheumatoid arthritics, tend to have numerous triggers, as do individuals with sluggish metabolism such as hypothyroid patients. A list of conditions in which trigger points are commonly found includes:

- osteoarthritis
- irritable bowel syndrome
- Crohn's Disease
- adrenal insufficiency
- migraine headaches
- slipped or herniated disc
- chronic candidiasis
- chronic hepatitis
- constipation
- hypothyroidism
- Epstein-Barr Syndrome
- tension headaches
- fibromyositis
- rheumatoid arthritis
- temporomandibular joint (TMJ) syndrome

How to Treat Trigger Points

Trigger points are localized regions of compression. They represent a concentration of forces due to factors such as muscular and ligamentous tension, vertebral displacement, injury, toxicity, edema, inflammation, and nerve tension/irritability. While pressing on the trigger may provide temporary or partial relief, the quickest, most effective method of treating them is decompression. This is accomplished by "popping" the trigger via the use of injections. Popping triggers is actually quite descriptive. It is common to hear a crunching or popping noise when these regions are injected. Usually, when the pop occurs, it is associated with a sudden, measurable reduction in pain. The headache itself may not disappear immediately. Yet, sometimes it does, and there is usually a certain degree of sustained relief from the pain. More important is the fact that trigger point injections act to gradually eliminate painful stimuli which result from irritated nerves, inflamed tissues, and tense muscles. By eliminating the sites of pain, an effective, long lasting cure can be achieved in a majority of cases.

The Technique

I was first introduced to this technique by an osteopathic physician, Hal Polance, D.O., of Cedar Rapids, Iowa. Dr. Polance is currently retired.

Many of Dr. Polance's patients were headache victims, whose headaches had been cured or reduced in severity via the injections. Patients would make appointments to request "the shot."

With time and experience I modified Dr. Polance's technique. The modified technique was even more effective than the aforementioned method for eradicating headaches as well as other forms of chronic pain. It was not until I attended a medical conference in Nevada that the scientific value of this modification came to light. There, a German physician gave a lecture about the science of *Neural Therapy*. Interestingly, Neural Therapy is the German equivalent to trigger point injections. Over the years the Germans found, as I have also determined through experience with my patients, that Neural Therapy works best if the injection is delivered immediately under the skin. The deeper the needle enters, the less pronounced is the response.

Most physicians would probably think that the needle must enter the deeper structures to deliver its medicine "on target." While this may be true of a cortisone shot into a joint, it couldn't be further from the truth regarding headache triggers. While a few injections need to be delivered at moderate depths of 1/8th of an inch or so, most should enter the skin no deeper than one millimeter. This means that, for optimum effect, the needle must be fixed just barely under the skin. Once the needle is fixed, the fluid should be injected until a wheel or circle is formed. This technique is similar to that used by allergists, who perform scratch testing.

Trigger points are most intensely painful during or just preceding a migraine. Often, they remain tender for a few days after the migraine subsides. Any of these situations are ideal times for trigger points to be injected.

What is injected?

The composition of the fluid that is injected depends on a number of factors. Nearly always, the principal constituent is *procaine*. Procaine is the same substance dentists use to numb teeth. It is a local anesthetic. It is commonly used by surgeons and emergency room doctors to numb injured tissue prior to suturing. A few people are allergic to local anesthetics of the *caine* family. These anesthetics include procaine (novocaine), carbocaine, and marcaine. Before administering the injections, it is important to ask if any known sensitivity or allergy to local anesthetics exists. If there is, other solutions devoid of local anesthetics must be utilized. The injection solution usually contains additional substances which influence nerve function and reduce cellular inflammation. These include vitamins B-12 and B-5 (pantothenic acid). The B-vitamins offer the added benefit of directly nourishing the nerves. B-12 by itself may be used with excellent results, as can a solution of sterile salt water. What matters more than the type of fluid is where and how it is injected.

How much is injected?

Only a very tiny needle is needed to infuse the fluid. This is a 30-gauge needle. The pain felt when the needle enters the skin is minimal. A small amount of fluid is injected, usually no more than 2/10ths of a cubic centimeter, just enough to pop, that is release, the trigger point and ease the pain. Usually, multiple sites are injected in one session.

The pain from the medicine and injection is rather mild. There are many types of pain that people experience of far greater severity. There is more pain involved in having blood drawn, and a cortisone shot can't compare. When contrasted to these, trigger point shots are a relatively painless experience.

Who can do it?

Only medically licensed physicians, D.O.'s and M.D.'s, can perform these injections. Unfortunately, only a few physicians in the United States are skilled in this technique.

Why trigger point therapy works

Dr. Harold Wolfe, a neurologist and author of the 800-page book, *Headache and Other Head Pain,* concluded after many years of research that in the majority of headaches pain arises from pain sensitive structures located superficially. He found that pain was concentrated in the outer layers of the scalp, the skin of the upper neck, the skin around the temples, the sinuses and the superficial veins, and arteries. He concluded that these tissues were ultrasensitive to pain, more so than intracranial ones. He also found the inflammation which occurred within the skull resulted in referred pain in these superficial regions. Even the deep pain which many chronic migraine sufferers experience was found to be due to irritation and inflammation of the superficial structures. Trigger point injections exert their effects on the most superficial components of headache pain. Through this action these injections help eliminate the acute pain of a headache crisis.

How do painful triggers arise?

All pain arises from highly complex interactions occurring within the central nervous system. Also known as the CNS, it is divided primarily into two sections: the brain and the spinal cord. The stimulus for pain often originates from a distance, for example, from a cut or bruise. Have you ever cut yourself without knowing it, only to feel pain seconds or minutes later? This is partly due to the time it takes for the injury to be evaluated and processed by the CNS. Once the CNS establishes the "need" for pain, it creates a pain reflex. This reflex is fixed within the spinal cord until the need for pain disappears. This means that until a cut heals, there will be pain. Until muscle spasms ease, there will be discomfort. Unfortunately, with migraine the pain reflex seems to become established more permanently. This pain cycle within the spinal cord remains intact, that is until it is broken either naturally or artificially. The cycle is involuntary, but things such as mind-set, meditation, manipulative treatment, pain medicines, and anti-inflammatory agents can break or diminish it. Yet, nothing seems so powerful in disrupting it as trigger point injections. Through accurate injection of triggers, the pain cycle is disengaged, often immediately. The stubborn spinal cord pain reflex seems to give up. There is usually an immediate sense of relief, as if a weight has been lifted from the head. Usually, the pain disappears within 24 to 48 hours. Ultimately, through repeated sessions, the spinal cord loses its memory for pain, and the trigger points disappear.

Precisely why the injection of trigger points relieves local or distant pain still remains unclear. However, the technique serves as a sensible, non-toxic solution to the seemingly insurmountable problem of chronic pain. It is a safer solution than medications, but more importantly, trigger point therapy targets the cause, something that medications rarely if ever do.

Chapter 7

Natural Cures

Herbal medicines, as well as nutritional supplements, are effective against migraines. Spices, which are normally regarded as mere foods, are also proving to be curative. Nutrients, that is vitamins, minerals, amino acids, and enzymes, have mild but significant anti-headache powers.

Nutrients tend to improve migraines by enhancing overall health and by increasing the body's resistance to stress as well as pain. Natural substances are a reliable alternative to drugs. Plus, they offer a significant benefit: the lack of side effects.

Vitamin-mineral therapy greatly increases the resistance to disease, and headaches are no exception. Whenever overall health is improved, this will aid in the reversal of all diseases, including migraines.

There are several categories of natural compounds which are beneficial for treating migraines. They include herbs, minerals, vitamins, amino acids, enzymes, and fatty acids. Each of these is described within this chapter.

Herbal Medicines

It is unfortunate that in some circles herbs have been given a negative connotation. Their use as therapeutic agents is often associated with extremism and quackery. Certainly, there may be herbal gurus who practice on the fringes. Yet, to condemn herbs per se as a result of the practices of the few would be foolish to say the least. The fact is herbs are safer than drugs, plus in many instances they are more effective. What's more, in contrast to drugs, herbs can, in fact, help the body in curing disease.

Herbs are valuable for the treatment of illness, and in some instances they are aggressive cures. As many as 80% of the drugs on the market are modeled after plant and herbal derivatives. These derivatives are known as *active ingredients*. These potent ingredients are responsible for the medicinal actions of herbs.

There are tens of thousands of herbs. Only a few have practical medicinal uses. It is easy to become confused by the plethora of herbs available, and, still, there are many thousands yet to be discovered. Few people, except scholars in botany, have a complete understanding of this chemistry and these medicinal properties.

The Chinese know a great deal about herbs. In fact, in China herbs are the main prescription for treating disease. Many Chinese doctors know more about herbs than they do about medications. This book will focus on herbs which are highly safe and which have been proven effective through scientific studies.

Herbs for Migraines

Relatively few herbs have been studied for anti-migraine activity. However, recently, a number of herbs have been touted. One of these is feverfew. In my experience it is relatively weak in reversing migraines. There is a word of caution: feverfew is botanically a weed, like a grass. Therefore, allergy to it may be common. The quality of feverfew products depends entirely upon the potency of the herbal extracts and the method of their preparation.

A favorite use of herbs and spices is a culinary one. It involves the heavy use of strong spices/herbs as flavoring agents and digestive aids. In this way herbs and, to some degree, spices may be helpful in preventing migraines. The exception would be those who are allergic to them, and this allergy would negate any beneficial effect.

It is easy to comprehend how spices help fight migraines as well as other types of headaches. In particular, spices are highly effective against sinus migraines. There are several mechanisms for such actions. Spices are top sources of magnesium, the anti-migraine mineral. This addition of magnesium into the diet can be considerable, depending upon how much and what type of spices are used. As tissue levels of magnesium rise, the propensity for migraine is decreased proportionately. In addition, hot spices are digestive stimulants. They also boost the metabolic rate, increasing the speed at which fats and sugars are burned as energy. Many herbs are fine sources of potassium which is an excellent nerve tonic. In addition, herbs, such as ginger and turmeric, contain potent anti-inflammatory compounds known as *flavonoids*. According to the latest research flavonoids are just as potent in reducing inflammation as many drugs.

Ginger is a case in point. It is a strong antidote for inflammations of the stomach and liver. Ginger is an effective remedy for migraines which are due to inflammation in these organs. For ginger to have a positive effect considerable amounts must be consumed either as fresh ginger or as a supplement.

Turmeric is another valuable antiinflammatory herb. This bright yellow substance is found in curry powder and is also used as a coloring for mustard. Turmeric can be taken in a supplemental form as a natural antiinflammatory agent. Other herbs and spices are listed as follows, along with the mechanism responsible for their positive effects.

Herb/Spice

- hot pepper ....improves circulation; speeds metabolic rate
- coriander ....one of the richest natural sources of potassium; reduces swelling
- garlic ....improves circulation; decreases platelet aggregation
- onion ....improves circulation; decreases platelet aggregation
- licorice root ....reduces inflammation; enhances adrenal function
- ginseng ....improves blood flow; enhances adrenal function
- rosemary ....improves blood flow to the brain; strengthens adrenals

When selecting herbs and spices, choose those which are prepared without radiation. Unfortunately, virtually all spices found in the grocery store have been irradiated. This leads to measurable levels of radioactivity within the spices. Do your part to boycott the use of nuclear waste to irradiate our food through buying only non-irradiated spices and herbs. These are available at fine health food stores. Hopefully, grocery stores will eventually carry them too. The more demand that is created for these quality edibles, the more likely it is that they will be made conveniently available everywhere.

Minerals

Mineral deficiency is common in migraineurs. However, do minerals really provide migraine relief? To comprehend this it is important to review the role played by minerals in human physiology.

Minerals are the stuff of life itself. Every plant is dependent upon them for survival. It is well known that the quality of the food supply is entirely dependent upon the health of the soil upon which it is grown, and the basis of the soil is minerals. Animals too must have minerals. In the wild they receive them from plants, other animals, and water. Some animals even chew on rocks, coal, or soil to get their minerals. Today, domesticated animals are given mineral supplements. Research and experience have determined that animals benefit from mineral-rich foods and supplements. Without these vital substances, animals fail to thrive. Wouldn't the same be true of man?

It is likely that the reader is mineral deficient. A person might respond by saying, "I eat a balanced diet and take a multiple vitamin/mineral supplement. I get all I need." This thinking is erroneous. Regardless of how well a person eats mineral deficiencies still exist. Commercially grown foods are mineral deficient, often severely so. Softened water is deficient. Reverse osmosis and distilled water are totally deficient. Processed foods are super-deficient. White flour, white rice, and, especially, white sugar are utterly devoid of minerals. Do you know anyone whose diet is completely free of these substances? Or, do you know anyone who eats exclusively organically grown foods, which are grown on composted, mineral-rich soil? Only such a person would be getting sufficient minerals.

How many people do you know who eat tree-ripened produce and organically raised meats? Few if any people eat this way. This is the kind of lifestyle one would have to follow to get a balanced amount of natural minerals.

Minerals are the spark plugs of the human engine. They act to fire-up chemical reactions. They assist in the maintenance of proper glandular and, therefore, hormone function. They help soothe and nourish the nerves and muscles.

It should be no surprise that symptoms such as fatigue, depression, and anxiety are often due to mineral deficiency. One way to discover the existence of mineral deficiency is to take the following exam:

Mineral Deficiency Exam

Which of the following applies to you?

Symptom/Condition	Deficient Mineral
1. leg cramps	Ca, Mg, K
2. toe or foot cramps	Ca, Mg, K
3. brittle or soft nails	Ca, Mg, K, Si, Fe, Zn
4. brittle bones (history of frequent fractures)	Ca, Cu, K, Si, Mn, Mg, Zn
5. history of anemia	Cu, Fe, K, Se
6. fatigue	Cr, K, Mg, Se, Zn
7. fall asleep after eating	Cr, K, Mg, Zn
8. white spots on fingernails	Zn
9. hang nails	Zn
10. irritable nerves	Ca, K, Mg, Na
11. high blood pressure	Ca, Cr, K, Mg, Mn, Zn
12. ridges on fingernails	Ca,, Mg, Si, Su
13. headaches	Cr, Ca, K, Mg
14. nerve twitching	Ca, K, Mg

15. constipation	K, Mg, Se
16. menstrual cramps	Ca, K, Mg
17. kidney stones	K, Mg
18. eczema or psoriasis	Ca, Zn
19. impaired sense of smell	Zn
20. elevated cholesterol or triglyceride	Cr, Mn, Se
21. depression	Ca, Cr, K, Mg
22. susceptible to allergy reactions	Ca, K, Se, Mo
23. cold extremities	Ca, K, Mg, Zn
24. hair loss or brittle hair	Cu, Si, Su, Zn
25. anxiety	Ca, Co, K, Mg
26. insomnia	Ca, Cr, K, Mg
27. stiffness of joints	Ca, Cu, K, Mg
28. blood sugar disturbances	Cr, K, Mg, Zn

KEY

Ca	Calcium	K	Potassium	Se	Selenium
Cr	Chromium	Mg	Magnesium	Si	Silicon
Co	Cobalt	Mn	Manganese	Su	Sulfur
Cu	Copper	Mo	Molybdenum	Zn	Zinc
Fe	Iron				

As this test demonstrates minerals are important for the maintenance of overall health. This function is more critical than any anti-migraine effect. Yet, certain minerals may help abort migraines, most notably calcium, magnesium, and chromium. What's more, the regular intake of such critical anti-migraine minerals is a significant component of any migraine-prevention strategy.

Calcium: The Nerve Tonic Mineral

Just why calcium helps prevent migraines is unknown. However, by reviewing its functions some light can be shed on the subject. Calcium is required for normal transmission of nerve impulses. Depending upon the dose it can act either to excite or sedate the nerves. In high doses, such as 2,000 or more mg daily, it acts more like a sedative. In other words, calcium relaxes the nervous system.

Huge doses of calcium, however, may not be a good idea. This may create a mineral imbalance, especially an imbalance of magnesium. Thus, the safest approach is to consume modest levels such as 1000 mg daily.

Ideally, calcium supplements should contain two other components: vitamin D and magnesium. In nature magnesium is usually found with calcium. Vitamin D is needed for the absorption of both these minerals. There is a word of caution: vitamin D can be toxic. No more than 8,000 I.U. should be taken on a daily basis. What's more, the maximum daily dose of calcium, that is for maintenance purposes, should be no more than 1500 mg. The best results with high dose calcium can be achieved by taking magnesium. This is because the latter mineral aids in both the absorption of calcium as well as its deposition in the bone. About 400 mg per day is a reasonable dose.

It is important to remember that most people, particularly women, lose calcium as they age. Women who smoke, drink, or take the Pill are especially at risk. Thus, certain women fail to consume sufficient calcium to maintain normal bone density. In addition, those who strictly avoid milk products usually have a calcium deficiency, that is unless they are taking supplements. The prescribed dosages will give the body a chance to build up calcium levels in the bones. This ultimately means that there is more calcium available to be drawn out of the bones whenever the body needs it. The result is a calm nervous system, and, thus, headaches are kept at bay.

It should be noted that many nutrients are involved in keeping the bones strong. Calcium alone is not sufficient. Also, many women are under the impression that estrogen, especially after menopause, is crucial for the maintenance of strong bones. It isn't as critical as some maintain. What is important is a balance of all the bone-building nutrients. Other bone-building minerals include zinc, copper, silicon, iodine, and manganese.

Bone is a living tissue and can be renewed. Bone tissue requires a steady supply of the nutrients it thrives on. Strong bones and joints are important in headache prevention. Weight bearing is a constant stress on the skeleton and spine. The more the skeleton can withstand the pressures of gravity—jars, tumbles, and mishaps of everyday life—the more resistant it will be to stress and trauma-induced headaches. Most migraine patients know that stress and structural problems can precipitate migraines. Keeping the spine strong is just one more preventive measure which can be taken.

People at extra risk for calcium deficiency headaches include:

- dialysis patients
- birth control pill users
- alcoholics
- those with a history of gastric stapling, gastric balloon, or intestinal bypass
- sugar addicts
- cigarette smokers
- coffee drinkers

Only a comparatively few foods are rich in calcium. In many of these the calcium is difficult to absorb. For example, spinach and sesame seeds contain calcium oxalate which is poorly absorbed and can even cause some toxicity. Contrary to popular belief, calcium in milk products is relatively easy to absorb and constitutes a substantial dietary source. A recent study showed that milk calcium is absorbed as well, if not better, than typical calcium supplemental sources such as egg or oyster shell. Top food sources of calcium include:

- canned salmon
- cheese (goat's or cow's milk)
- milk
- cream
- fermented milk products
- scallops
- shrimp
- herring
- sardines
- mackerel
- dark green vegetables, especially watercress, parsley, and broccoli
- nuts, especially almonds

Fish are listed, because when canned, the bones are included. These bones dissolve and can be chewed. The calcium may then be absorbed. Fermented milk products are an excellent calcium source. The fermentation process makes the calcium easier to absorb. Acid assists calcium transport into the blood.

Allergy to milk products is a significant problem in migraine sufferers, and this may create difficulties in achieving adequate intake of dietary calcium. In this instance other food sources of calcium must be regularly consumed. Watercress is one of the top vegetable sources, containing more calcium by weight than milk products. However, as with any other vegetable source it must be well chewed or, preferably, juiced so that the calcium can be liberated for absorption. Carrot juice is also rich in absorbable calcium. However, it is high in sugar and, thus, may be poorly tolerated by headache sufferers, especially those with hypoglycemia. Other excellent vegetable sources of calcium include wild oregano, wild rosemary, turnip and beet greens, mustard greens, dill weed, parsley, and basil. Nuts are an excellent source, particularly almonds and hazelnuts. Other top sources of calcium include sardines, dried figs, trout (canned), salmon (canned), and poppy seeds.

Certain spices/herbs are top calcium sources. This includes basil, rosemary, thyme, and wild oregano. Of these wild oregano is perhaps supreme. Wild oregano capsules have proven effective in regenerating bone density. Wild oregano grows on calcium-rich rock, even white marble. Thus, OregaMax (NAHS Co), the original high-density wild oregano formula, is the ideal natural calcium supplement, since it contains the type of minerals which are easy to absorb. Since it is the crude herb, to get a sufficient dose several capsules are needed, usually six to eight daily. In the event of severe bone loss or joint disorders take up to 12 daily. Bone densitometry proves that the type of calcium and magnesium in crude wild oregano capsules is fully incorporated into bone, better than the type in the typical calcium tablet. Instead of difficult-to-digest hard calcium pills, OregaMax offers natural "homeopathic" doses of calcium, which are readily used by the body. There are no digestive disturbances or side effects with it. Rather, it aids digestion.

Magnesium: Migraine Blocking Agent?

Magnesium is the second most abundant mineral in the body. It serves several critical functions including maintenance of healthy nerves, muscles, joints, and bones.

Magnesium deficiency is common and affects more than half the population. This is largely a result of the fact that the soils upon which our food is grown are magnesium deficient. It is also because processed foods contain little or no magnesium. Raw sugar pressed from the cane is rich in magnesium, but refined sugar contains none. Fresh ground whole wheat flour is an excellent source; but with white flour, some 80% of the original magnesium is lost in the refining process. The loss of this mineral in canned vegetables is over 80%, and frozen vegetables rapidly lose magnesium in the water in which they are boiled. Soft and distilled water contain no appreciable amounts. Drinking these types of water leads to magnesium deficiency. The same dilemma may result from drinking water treated by reverse osmosis. Mineral water rich in magnesium or purified tap water would be healthier sources.

Magnesium plays an important role as a spark plug for our cells. This spark plug action is most pronounced in the nervous system where magnesium is responsible for the initiation of nerve impulses. It is also required for contraction and relaxation of the muscles. Magnesium deficiency can lead to nerve irritability and muscular tension. In fact, when magnesium deficiency is pronounced, the muscles often become so tense that they are easily injured or torn.

Scientific evidence supports the use of magnesium in the treatment of migraines. Recent studies by doctors at the University of Tennessee showed that supplemental magnesium in a dose of 200 milligrams per day brought significant migraine relief, particularly in women. Some 80% of the women tested found their migraines to be completely gone shortly after beginning the supplements. Magnesium was so effective that it was used to stop migraines once they occurred. Many of the subjects discovered that if they took magnesium within half an hour of the migraine onset, the symptoms would abate entirely.

Migraine patients should take magnesium on a daily basis. The typical maintenance dosage would be 200 to 500 milligrams per day. An excellent, highly absorbable magnesium is manufactured by Nutritiontest.com Formulas under the brand name, *Magnesium Chelate*. This type of magnesium is highly recommended, since it is less likely to cause digestive upset than many other brands. Magnesium is difficult to absorb. When too much magnesium enters the intestines at one time, diarrhea and cramping result. This problem appears to be eliminated by the use of amino acid chelates. One of the best is magnesium taurate. The latter stands for *taurine*, an amino acid to which the magnesium is bound. Taurine helps carry magnesium into the cells, keeping it from irritating the gut due to a lack of absorption. In fact, it is the body's naturally occurring magnesium transportation system.

Many drugs cause magnesium deficiency. A partial list includes:

- antibiotics
- digitalis
- alcohol
- calcium channel blockers
- aspirin
- diuretics
- cortisone
- laxatives

In particular, diuretics aggressively deplete this mineral. For those taking diuretic drugs regular supplementation with a high grade magnesium supplement is essential. A minimum of 400 mg per day must be taken.

Spices, especially hot ones, and also nuts, seeds, whole grains, soybeans, dark green leafy vegetables, and cocoa, are rich dietary sources of magnesium. Did you see that last item—cocoa? Yes, cocoa is an excellent magnesium source, being one of the top ten sources known. Could the chocolate cravings of migraine patients be nothing more than instinctual desires to correct underlying magnesium deficiencies? It is likely, especially if these cravings occur in women around their menstrual periods, since magnesium is depleted during menses.

Chromium: Blood Sugar Regulating Mineral

Chromium is another mineral useful in the prevention of migraines. One of its most critical functions is to help drive sugar—blood glucose—into the brain. Research has shown that glucose enters brain cells up to four times more efficiently when chromium is supplemented in the diet. The brain needs extra glucose as the result of stress. Chromium may help reduce the length or severity of a migraine, especially if the migraine is due to hypoglycemia and/or emotional stress.

When people think of chromium, they often think of chrome, the metal found on car bumpers. There is no comparison with natural chromium. Inorganic chromium is very difficult to absorb. Thus, while chrome is made up of atoms of chromium, the way it exists molecularly makes absorption impossible. However, as has been borne out by numerous scientific studies, organically bound chromium is more easily absorbed than the inorganic type.

There are several excellent chromium supplements on the market. The names include yeast-bound chromium, glucose tolerance factor, chromium picolinate, and chromium nicotinate. All these products are of value. Chromium picolinate and nicotinate are yeast-free, which is important in certain cases of allergic migraine. Plus, measurable, predictable responses result when these two formulations are used therapeutically. A standard dosage is 100 to 200 micrograms three times daily.

Because chromium is found in so few foods, the only reasonable way to get it is via a supplement. This is true unless one is a connoisseur of rice bran or brewer's yeast. If consumed regularly both of these foods suffice as chromium supplements. Other good sources of chromium include organ meats, wheat germ, and whole grains.

There is a natural form of chromium, strictly from food. This is in the form of crude grape extract from mountain-grown red sour grapes. The red grapes concentrate chromium from the soil. Crude red grape extract, known commercially as Resvitanol, contains virtually the highest concentration of chromium of any natural substance. A mere teaspoon of this raw natural product contains as much as 40% of the minimum requirement. For people who are sensitive to chemical-based supplements Resvitanol is ideal. A typical dosage is a teaspoon twice daily. Crude red grape offers yet another benefit: improved blood flow. This can be invaluable for headache sufferers. Blood flow is impaired in headache sufferers. The regular intake of Resvitanol reverses this. The fact is the crude red grape helps regenerate the entire arterial system. Thus, it is of exceptional value for migraine patients, who suffer from chronic arterial damage.

If you have migraines, be sure to build up your body levels of nerve-nourishing minerals. It may take as long as six months to replenish these levels. Taking the mentioned nutritional supplements would help, and a multiple vitamin/mineral supplement may also be necessary. However, men and post-menopausal women should avoid multiple vitamin/mineral supplements containing iron. The extra iron is not needed unless one is anemic, and it may even be harmful. Because of this, many companies offer multiple vitamin/mineral supplements which are iron free.

Vitamins

There is no scientific evidence that vitamins relieve migraines. Most vitamins are weak in terms of anti-migraine effect.

However, vitamins are important for the maintenance of overall health, and, in this regard, all vitamins are important in relation to the migraine problem. A few vitamins play an exceptional role in migraine physiology. They are pantothenic acid, vitamin B-6 (pyridoxine), vitamin C, and vitamin E. By looking at the mechanism of action of these vitamins, their value in the treatment of the migraine patient is revealed.

Riboflavin: Cellular Oxygenator

The brain is the body's greatest consumer of oxygen. Riboflavin facilitates this process. This substance is perhaps more a coenzyme than a vitamin. Riboflavin is directly involved in oxygen metabolism. It is an essential component of a special cellular process known as the respiratory chain. This is a chain of enzymes which process fuel, that is glucose, into energy. Oxygen is needed for this processing. Riboflavin is required for the oxygen to be metabolized. Without it, the entire process comes to a halt. The fact is riboflavin is the essential nutrient for proper oxygen utilization by the cells. This is particularly true of the brain, where this vitamin helps the neurons process both oxygen and fuel.

Recently, researchers determined that migraine sufferers are largely riboflavin deficient. Thus, they gave the vitamin, about 50 mg per day. Incredibly, the migraines improved some 50%. Thus, a daily dose of riboflavin can prove highly valuable in the cure of this condition. What's more, natural sources of riboflavin are invaluable. One of the top sources is a wild greens supplement, the Cell-u-clenz Powerdrops. These drops are made from wild forest and meadow greens, notably wild dandelion, nettles, and burdock. A top source of naturally occurring riboflavin, the wild greens have helped a number of individuals in reversing or halting headache symptoms, including pain, pressure, fatigue, and nausea. The Powerdrops are rare. Only a limited supply is available. Unavailable at most stores they must be ordered by calling 1-800-243-5242. In Canada call 1-866-drspice (1-866-776-6550). The riboflavin content is about one milligram per ounce, which is incredibly high for a natural product. Other natural sources of this vitamin include egg yolks, liver, red meat, fish, dark green leafy vegetables, bee pollen, raw honey, royal jelly, and fatty fish. Thus, people on low-fat and vegetable-based diets are at a high risk for riboflavin deficiency.

Pantothenic Acid: Vitamin Powerhouse

Few vitamins exert as potent a biological effect as pantothenic acid. The use of pantothenic acid during a migraine may occasionally be of value, but its main use is as a tonic for the adrenal glands. This vitamin strengthens these glands and normalizes hormone synthesis. Thus, it boosts the ability of the adrenal glands to fight stress. This is the primary means by which pantothenic acid can aid the headache victim.

Regular supplementation with pantothenic acid can reduce the frequency and severity of hypoglycemia-induced headaches. Also, the adrenals will be more capable of warding off allergy reactions, reducing the likelihood of an allergy-induced migraine. Research has proven that moderate-to-high doses of pantothenic acid can induce the synthesis of adrenal steroids. These extra steroids help prevent allergy reactions, reduce inflammation, and keep blood sugar levels stable. As stated previously weakened or over-stressed adrenals are unable to maintain proper blood sugar levels. Thus, even a seemingly slight stress, such as failing to eat breakfast or the aggravation of being stuck in traffic, can bring on a headache. The brain must receive sufficient glucose, since this nutrient is its primary food. A sudden drop in blood sugar levels often affects the brain, and this is manifested by mental symptoms. Here is where pantothenic acid plays one of its most critical roles. It can cause a rapid increase in the production and secretion of adrenal hormones. Once these hormones enter the bloodstream, blood sugar levels are normalized.

The recommended dosage may vary, depending upon the severity of stress or the headache history. A typical maintenance dose is 500 milligrams three times daily. This should be taken in conjunction with B-complex supplements, as the B-vitamins work best if all are available to the tissues at the same time. Up to three grams can be taken daily with no known toxicity. However, there is one negative result from taking such high doses: the inside of the nose can become dry. If you notice this, the dosage should be reduced, although there are no long-term ill effects of this dryness. Yet, obviously, the ideal source of this vitamin is natural sources, which are completely non-toxic.

Excellent pantothenic acid supplements are made by several companies. Some of these companies make time-released products. In the case of pantothenic acid time-released is good, since this vitamin can be absorbed throughout the intestinal tract. This is not true of many other B-vitamins. An excellent formulation is made by Cardiovascular Research and is called Pantothene. This is a special form of pantothenic acid. Pantothene is of exceptional value, since it can be taken in high doses with less risk of toxicity. This is important during a migraine crisis when high doses of pantothenic acid may be useful. In addition, studies show that supplementation with Pantothene leads to improved circulation by inhibiting platelet adherence, a phenomenon which contributes to migraine pathology. Yet, there is a way to get the pantothenic acid from natural sources: unprocessed royal jelly. The fact is royal jelly is the top naturally occurring source of this vitamin. Royal Kick is a highly potent form of royal jelly, superior to the commercial type. It provides microdoses of natural-source royal jelly, which greatly aids body functions. For people with sensitive systems who fail to tolerate synthetic vitamins this is the ideal source. As a natural source of pantothenic acid take three capsules twice daily.

Vitamin B6: Nature's Diuretic

Vitamin B-6 is an important migraine prevention agent. This vitamin has a natural diuretic action, stimulating the kidneys to excrete excess water. Allergy reactions cause water retention and can even lead to the accumulation of water in the brain. B-6 exerts its diuretic action most profoundly when combined with essential fatty acids such as GLA or crude pumpkinseed oil (Pumpkinol).

B-6 is involved in other important functions relative to migraine. These involve the synthesis of brain chemicals known as neurotransmitters. Along with magnesium, B-6 is required for the synthesis and function of these neurological chemicals. Care must be taken in "megadose" B-6 therapy, since it could lead to toxicity. An excellent, non-toxic form of B-6 is available. It is called P-5-P, which stands for pyridoxal-5-phosphate. A way to avoid B-6 toxicity is to take 50 to 100 milligrams of P-5-P whenever taking more than 100 milligrams of regular B-6. By doing this higher doses can be taken with safety. However, such dosages should not exceed 500 milligrams per day. The exceptions are certain rare diseases involving genetic defects.

Vitamin C: The Natural Antihistamine

Vitamin C is a powerhouse vitamin. It helps prevent allergic reactions by boosting immune defenses. It strengthens the adrenal glands and is required for the synthesis of all adrenal hormones. Vitamin C is Nature's antihistamine. With all these functions, vitamin C helps block the allergic reactions which lead to migraines.

Histamine is a major player in allergic reactions. It is a natural chemical, which is released in large quantities from certain types of white blood cells, known as mast cells, as a consequence of allergic reactions. Migraine headaches, being primarily allergic in origin, are associated with increased histamine levels. Histamine itself, if injected into the body, can provoke migraines in susceptible individuals. For these reasons it is important to prevent histamine levels from rising. Vitamin C, as crude natural vitamin C, is found in the supplement Flavin-C. This is made exclusively from natural ingredients. Taken on a daily basis Flavin-C is an ideal antihistaminic agent. It also helps boost adrenal function, and it is the adrenal glands which fight allergic reactions. Thus, by regularly supplying these glands with their needed dose of natural vitamin C, allergic propensities are reduced, perhaps eliminated.

Vitamin E: Blood Flow Performer

For years it has been known that vitamin E exerts many of its beneficial effects by improving blood flow. However, there is little evidence that vitamin E relieves migraines. Vitamin E does increase the ability of the blood to carry oxygen. It acts as a natural blood thinner and improves the ability of the heart to pump blood. Vitamin E also upgrades the immune response and is an anti-inflammatory agent.

Even though it is fat soluble, vitamin E is one of the safest vitamins known. Thus, it can be taken in high doses without toxicity. There is one exception. Certain people with high blood pressure must proceed with caution when taking vitamin E. With dosages higher than 400 I.U. blood pressure may be raised. However, in most instances taking vitamin E during a headache can only help. Yet, there are totally natural ways to get vitamin E. This is through low dose sources such as certain foods, food oils, and food-like supplements. Crude pumpkinseed oil, known as Pumpkinol, is an ideal source of low-dose natural vitamin E.

There is no possibility of heightened blood pressure with this source. Rather, Pumpkinol helps lower it. As a natural source of the full vitamin E complex take two or more tablespoons daily.

Some people are allergic to soy. Thus, they are concerned they might be allergic to vitamin E made from soy oil. This can be a problem, but most soy allergies are to soy protein. Even so, the vitamin E, as well as soy oil, may be contaminated due to genetic engineering. This may lead to serious allergic reactions. Vitamin E comes from the oil. However, wheat germ oil is used in some vitamin E preparations, and wheat-sensitive individuals need to avoid such products. Previous experiences with patients have proven that wheat allergic individuals can get a migraine from consuming wheat germ oil or vitamin E products containing it. This is another reason to rely on Pumpkinol, since allergic intolerance to pumpkinseed oil is utterly rare.

Amino Acids

When most people think of nutrients, they think primarily of vitamins and minerals. This is understandable. It has been taught that vitamins and minerals are essential and that we must get them via the diet to remain healthy. However, there is another group of essential nutrients: the amino acids.

Over 30 amino acids exist, although only eight are classified as "essential." By definition, essential means that the nutrient cannot be made within the human body and, therefore, must be obtained via dietary sources. For example, the human body is incapable of synthesizing calcium, nor can it make the amino acid *phenylalanine*. Some vitamins can be synthesized, but the majority are essential, since they must be received through diet or from supplements.

Amino acids are derived from proteins that can be digested to yield the amino acids. These are then formulated into supplements. Amino acids may also be derived through bacterial fermentation.

The essential amino acids include the following:

- isoleucine
- leucine
- lysine
- methionine
- phenylalanine
- threonine
- tryptophan
- valine

Phenylalanine and tryptophan are probably the most important migraine-fighting amino acids. Tryptophan is nearly impossible to find. It was pulled off the market as a result of a serious illness which was associated with its use. A Japanese company is responsible for sending a contaminated batch of tryptophan to the United States. It was contaminated with a bizarre protein made by bacteria. The protein was produced by genetically engineered bacteria. This contaminant is the likely culprit behind a disorder known as *Eosinophillic Myalgic Syndrome* (EMS). This disorder sickened some 50,000 people, killing hundreds, perhaps thousands. Tryptophan itself is relatively non-toxic. People are now afraid of using tryptophan, and, to a degree, this is understandable. However, this is also unfortunate. Tryptophan has cured many cases of insomnia, PMS, and, yes, some cases of chronic pain and/or migraine. Whether tryptophan will ever be cleared by the FDA to be placed back on the market remains to be seen.

The tryptophan scare need not destroy confidence in the other amino acids, especially anti-pain ones such as leucine, tyrosine, and phenylalanine. Be sure to request from the manufacturer proof that the amino acids are non-GMO derived.

Phenylalanine is a case in point. As a supplement it can prove invaluable for controlling chronic pain. The DL form, known as DLPA, is the most common type available. DLPA is a natural pain modifier. It acts within the nervous system to control pain. Here is how this works. The brain naturally contains anti-pain compounds similar to opium, known as endorphins. Incredibly, these natural substances are up to 100 times more powerful than the drugs. This means that the human brain has its own painkilling mechanism which, if properly operating, could obliterate severe pain. The compounds, as discussed previously, are called endorphins and enkephalins. Researchers have discovered that, while endorphins and enkephalins are extremely powerful, their painkilling effects are limited by the fact that they are rapidly destroyed. The culprit appears to be an enzyme which inactivates endorphin and enkephalin molecules. This is where DLPA proves invaluable. It blocks the ability of the enzyme to deactivate these molecules. This results in a measurable rise in the endorphin/enkephalin levels within the central nervous system.

Chronic pain is commonly associated with endorphin/ enkephalin deficiency. In migraine patients, the levels of these substances may be severely depressed. DLPA is by no means a replacement for pain medicines. Its positive effects are gradual, and it may take up to three weeks before benefits are noticed. Yet, it is usually worth the wait. Studies have determined that over 75% of subjects improved in a wide variety of symptoms ranging from pain to depression. The ideal dosage appears to be 1 to 2 grams taken in divided doses.[1] If you are concerned about overdosing, consider this: DLPA is far less toxic than many of the pills commonly consumed *without concern* including antacids, aspirin, antihistamines, Motrin, Tylenol, and laxatives.

Tyrosine Prevents Hormone and Neurotransmitter Deficiency

Tyrosine is an important amino acid although not so much for its anti-pain effects. Its value is a result of the critical role it plays in human physiology. Tyrosine is the precursor for the

---

[1]Warning: Individuals with the hereditary condition phenylketonuria must avoid all nutritional supplements containing phenylalanine.

synthesis of hormones without which human life would be impossible: thyroxine and adrenaline. Without tyrosine, neither can be produced.

Tyrosine is needed to make thyroid hormone. Without it the production of this hormone halts. Adrenaline is produced in the adrenal glands. It also is produced from tyrosine. The thyroid gland is located in the front of the neck, just beneath the Adam's apple. The adrenal glands are located on top the kidneys. It is virtually assured that anyone who has a problem with thyroid and/or adrenal function also has a tyrosine deficiency. Furthermore, the brain produces adrenaline and also a compound known as noradrenaline (norepinephrine), both of which are derived from tyrosine. A deficiency of either of these neuro-transmitters increases the vulnerability of the nervous system to painful stimuli. Neurotransmitter deficiency has been associated with chronic pain syndromes, depression, anxiety, insomnia, and fatigue.

Boosting neurotransmitter levels is a major aid in fighting pain syndromes. This may be achieved through taking supplemental amino acids, such as tyrosine or phenylalanine, and by increasing the consumption of foods rich in these amino acids. Foods rich in amino acids include:

• beef	• fish
• lamb	• eggs
• organ meats	• yogurt
• poultry	• bee pollen
• cheese	• sesame seeds
• milk	• wild game

Tyrosine is one of the best nutritional cures for depression. This is because the amino acid helps increase brain levels of several neurotransmitters. Two have been mentioned; another is dopamine, a major mood-controlling chemical. Dopamine helps control a wide range of functions, including energy production and hormone secretion. Dopamine deficiency is relatively common. Severe stress or toxicity readily depletes it. This is what happens in Parkinson's disease, and the lack of dopamine is partly responsible for the severe rigidity these patients suffer.

Tyrosine is the key component of adrenaline. It helps replenish adrenaline levels within the adrenal glands after stress, because stress rapidly depletes adrenaline. One study showed that tyrosine enhances the body's ability to ward off allergic reactions. Thus, for individuals who are depressed, irritable, fatigued, and allergic, tyrosine may well be the answer. Tyrosine is a key component of the supplement ThyroAid.

Enzymes

Enzymes are complex protein molecules which serve as the body's work horses. Nearly every chemical process within living organisms depends upon enzymes. The life and function of plants is also entirely dependent upon the enzymes they contain.

A deficiency of enzymes or impaired enzyme function is a contributing factor to many illnesses. The extent of the negative effects depends upon how the enzyme fits into human biochemistry. If a deficiency of digestive enzymes occurs, food is improperly digested which increases the risk for allergic reactions. Incompletely digested food also contributes to the cause of many diseases, including arthritis, colitis, hypoglycemia, lupus, schizophrenia, psoriasis, eczema, diabetes and migraines. It may be necessary for individuals afflicted with these diseases to use digestive enzyme supplements. Often, this will cause a dramatic improvement in the symptoms. Digestion is a key to such a wide range of illnesses that it would be accurate to claim that virtually any condition will improve if digestion is enhanced.

A person's diet has a direct impact upon the cause of ill health. Improper diet directly impacts digestion. This is where enzymes are of value. They help normal digestion as well as cleanse the gut of toxins. Digestive enzymes may be the missing link between digestive impairment and the promotion of excellent overall health.

Enzymes serve a vast array of functions in the human body. In addition to normalizing digestion, they also act as a sort of garbage disposal system. In other words, they help clean up the cellular wastes. Debris, such as dead cells, tumors, and undigested foods, are made up primarily of protein. The only substances that can break down protein are enzymes. Enzymes act in a sense like miniature "pac men," gobbling up the dead protein, that is the dead cells or cellular waste. Under normal circumstances only dead and diseased tissue is attacked, while healthy tissue is immune to the enzymes' powers.

Enzymes assist the immune system in destroying foreign invaders. Bacteria, viruses, parasites, and yeasts are made up primarily of protein. White blood cells contain a considerable amount of enzymes. They use them to digest the microbe once they are engulfed.

It has been discovered that enzymes which are ingested in food can be absorbed into the bloodstream. For years it was believed that this was impossible. The previous thinking was that enzyme molecules are too large to be absorbed or that they, being made of protein, were completely destroyed by stomach acid. However, numerous scientific studies have proven that enzymes can be absorbed intact and that they are still biologically active. Could it be that the actual cells of the human body will incorporate and utilize these dietary and supplemental enzymes? That is the direction science is pointing.

Enzymes, Allergy, and Migraine

Enzymes can be useful in the treatment of migraines by improving digestion, thereby decreasing allergic tendencies. This has been known since the 1930s, when Dr. Oelgoetz, an M.D., found that pancreatic enzyme supplements significantly reduced food allergy-related symptoms. He published his findings in several medical journals. One of the allergy symptoms was migraine. In all cases migraines improved as a result of the enzyme therapy.

When using supplemental enzymes, some caution should be exerted. Pork allergy and, to a lesser degree, beef allergy are fairly common. Therefore, one might wish to utilize a less allergenic source such as lamb pancreas or vegetable source enzymes. Vegetable enzymes include those made from certain fungi, papain from papayas and also bromelain, which is derived from pineapples. There are a wide range of vegetable-source enzyme products available. One unique product is a combination of wild spices, aromatic herbs, and potent digestive enzymes. The wild spices, notably the wild oregano extract, destroy noxious germs, which disturb digestion, while the aromatic herbs calm the gut. The enzymes greatly boost digestive powers, stimulating the processing and assimilation of nutrients. The enzymes in this combination are fruit- and vegetable-based. This is a potent formula for reversing common digestive complaints, as demonstrated by the following:

CASE HISTORY:
Mr. C. is a 48-year-old male, who suffered a sudden case of indigestion due to contaminated food. He attempted the common remedies to no avail. Then, he was given a spice/enzyme concentrate. Within minutes after taking two capsules all the indigestion was relieved.

Note: For more information call: 1-800-243-5242

Migraten: Main Supplement for Headaches

It has been well known in the Third World for years that people who regularly eat hot spicy foods rarely get headaches. The more hot or pungent the herbs and spices, the more effective it is in reversing or preventing headache symptoms. Perhaps it is related to their antiinflammatory powers. Perhaps it is related to their positive effects upon circulation or their germicidal action. Pungent spices and herbs are the basis of Migraten.

Doctors realize that few if any pills can aggressively halt headaches. However, if the mechanism which causes headaches is reversed, the benefits can be major. Whenever the cause is treated, significant improvement, even cure, must occur. With migraines in particular a wide range of mechanisms must be addressed, and treatment must be aimed at all causes. This can be achieved by combining the powers of numerous herbs and spices which, in fact, help normalize the various imbalances. Migraten is such a formulation. This is a combination of potent herbs and spices, including wild rosemary, oregano, and basil, as well as ginger, each of which acts upon a different mechanism of migraine causation. Exceptionally powerful it reverses migraines as well as tension, stress, and cluster headaches. The subject of over 15 years of research, clinical investigations prove that Migraten is highly effective for virtually any type of headache, particularly migraines. One study by a clinician determined that this formula reduced the severity, as well as incidence, of headaches in all twelve subjects studied. This is largely due to this formula's potent analgesic and antiinflammatory powers. Migraten works within minutes. The fact is, usually, within an hour a massive improvement is noted, as is demonstrated by the following:

CASE HISTORY:

Mr. E. is a 33-year-old salesman, who suffers from day-long headaches. His headaches created pressure similar to a band around the head. The Migraten was taken, two capsules with water. Within fifteen minutes he noticed significant relief. Within two hours after taking four capsules the headache, as well as the tight sensation about his head, disappeared.

Migraten also addresses the hormonal factor. It contains a potent form of royal jelly, which helps normalize adrenal function. This helps stabilize blood sugar levels, which surely helps prevent headaches. In addition, it contains herbs and spices which help stabilize thyroid function. This, combined with its digestive-boosting capacity, as well as its potent antiinflammatory properties, demonstrates that Migraten is a complete complex for aggressively reversing headache pain. What's more, since it helps eradicate the cause the fact is Migraten may assist in the cure of headache syndromes.

The wild spice content of this formula is significant. Various spice extracts offer potent painkilling properties. This is due to their rich content of antiinflammatory phenols, including eugenol, rosmarinic acid, carvacrol, and thymol. A study performed in Turkey demonstrated the value of this effect. It was determined that a special type of wild oregano (the type used in Migraten) halted pain equally as well as many drugs and was nearly as powerful in painkilling power as morphine. This is why many people report migraine relief from taking edible oil of wild oregano. The fact is, oil of oregano is highly effective against migraine headaches. This is particularly true when the oil is taken under the tongue. Thus, wild herbs and spices offer potent support in pain syndromes, far more so than mere vitamins and minerals. What's more, these are herbs/spices which possess multiple medicinal actions. They ease digestive stress, combat allergic reactions, halt inflammation, strengthen the adrenals, boost thyroid function, and ease pain. Thus, they address the entire gamut of disorders: the inflammation, blood flow disorders, maldigestion, toxicity, allergic intolerance, and other syndromes responsible for headaches.

The antioxidant action of the herbs/spices in Migraten is notable. Rich in potent phenols, including the highly active compound rosmarinic acid, the components of Migraten help stabilize brain cells, preventing toxic damage. What's more, such antioxidants help preserve and stabilize cells in general, aiding in overall health. Thus, there is an anti-aging action of such a formula. There is another action in Migraten which, in fact, is a bonus: its effect upon brain function. With components such as royal jelly, wild rosemary, and wild St. John's wort, Migraten has vast actions upon brain chemistry, boosting mood and enhancing memory. The fact is depression, as well as memory loss, is a common consequence of chronic headaches. Regarding chronic migraines brain cell damage has been documented, including oxidative damage of the brain's arteries. This is why Migraten is invaluable. It not only helps eradicate headaches but also helps reverse any damage resulting from this disease.

How to use Migraten

Migraten is one of the most potent herb and spice formulas known. It has an aggressive action against head pain. The fact is it acts upon a variety of mechanisms related to the cause of headaches. Migraten contains potent antiinflammatory substances, as well as certain herbs, notably ginger, which balance digestive health. It is useful for all types of headaches. Simply take one or two capsules at the onset of a headache and repeat as needed, as often as on the hour. Ideally, always take it with food or juice. If nauseated, take smaller amounts, like a half capsule in juice or water as often as needed until symptoms are resolved. Also, take it preventively. One capsule daily is highly effective in preventing the onset of headaches, especially migraines. The regular daily intake of this formula will greatly reduce the severity and incidence of headaches and will likely cause their eradication.

However, for tough circumstances frequency is the key. It may be necessary to take it on the hour, in fact, every half hour. When taking such large amounts, it is recommended to take it with food or juice. Here is the typical dosage for eradicating a tough migraine: one or two capsules every hour or half hour until the pain disappears. With such high doses be sure to take Migraten with a small amount of food or tomato, grapefruit, or V-8 juice. This is the individual's first choice regarding effective migraine/headache cures. Ideally, Migraten must always be taken with food: for instance, a handful of nuts or a piece of meat or cheese, or plenty of fluids. As it is mainly a high potency spice extract this will help the extract disperse, so that it is non-irritating. As long as it is taken with food and/or fluids it is well tolerated. For those with a sensitive system even a half capsule is active: open the capsule and add half to tomato, V-8, or carrot juice. It may also be easily blended in fatty foods, for instance, whole milk, creamy cheeses, guacamole, nut butter, and extra virgin olive oil.

Migraten is the first choice in anti-headache supplements. The results with patients are highly positive. The oil of wild oregano, that is the P73 Oreganol, is also invaluable. This is because spice extracts destroy noxious germs, while eradicating pain and inflammation. Plus, spice extracts clear clogged sinuses. Recent evidence indicates that chronic infections, particularly of the sinus cavities, are a major factor in headaches. This is manifested by severe facial or head pain, often behind the eye or temple. The Migraten, as well as the oil of wild Oreganol, eliminates such symptoms, largely by destroying the germs. This demonstrates yet another mechanism regarding how spice extracts relieve, in fact, cure, headaches.

Migraten has proven equally as powerful in reversing headaches as any drug—without the side effects. This is no mere nutritional formula, rather, it is a combination of potent herbal and spice extracts with significant anti-inflammatory and anti-pain powers. Use it on a regular basis to prevent and eradicate headaches.

Fish Oils: Another Critical Supplement

It seems inconceivable that fats or oils could help cure migraines. Some believe that fats have derogatory effects, especially against the circulation. However, some fats actually improve circulation. The most dominating of these are the fish oils. These are known chemically as EPA and DHA.

The brain readily absorbs fish oils. Normally, EPA and DHA are found in brain and nerve tissue. In the Western diet fish oils are lacking, which upsets brain chemistry. Increasing the intake of fish oils, or fatty fish, can help normalize the brain circuitry.

Fish oils are potent anti-inflammatory agents. Thus, they function to prevent inflammation from occurring in nerve and brain tissue. The retina absorbs fish oils and the oils play a significant role in normal vision. Of all organs in the human body it appears that the brain has the greatest need for such oils. Mother was right about it being good for the brain.

The exact function of fish oils in the human brain is unknown. They do act as membrane stabilizers. This is important, since unstable nerve tissue increases the vulnerability for the development of illness, pain or inflammation.

These findings have astounding implications with regard to disorders of the nervous system. The inference is that brain tissue rich in fish oils is more stable against noxious stimuli which might damage or irritate the central nervous system. Could this also mean that the same stimulus which would have provoked a migraine no longer will if the brain contains a higher percentage of fatty acids from fish oils? Only further research will tell.

Fish oils exert several other positive effects upon the circulatory system. They help improve blood flow, and this effect can be dramatic. They assist in the healing of damaged arterial walls and prevent healthy ones from degenerating. Hardening of the arteries, a plague of modern civilization, is non-existent in Eskimos who eat fatty fish. Fish oils prevent blood clots, thereby diminishing the incidence of stroke, and they virtually eliminate sludging of the blood. Such sludging is obvious in migraines as well as in lung disease, heart disease, claudication, high blood pressure, Raynaud's disease, diabetes, and peripheral vascular disease.

Fish oils are Nature's blood thinners par excellence. They are superior in this action over aspirin, without the side effects. This blood thinning effect is easy to explain. It appears that the platelets, the cells responsible for blood clotting, have a preference for EPA and DHA similar to that seen in brain cells. Platelets rapidly incorporate fish oils into their membranes. The oils somehow alter platelet function to keep them from becoming excessively sticky. Having sticky platelets can be a dangerous thing, especially if there is a family history or a current history of circulatory disease, blood clots or stroke.

These various actions are why fish oils are one of the top anti-migraine nutrients. Science is proving this. Researchers have found that during the migraine crisis, fish oils reduce the inflammation of migraines. In the proper dose these oils lessen the severity of migraine attacks by 50%. Just think what can be accomplished preventively by religiously consuming fish oils every day. The result will undoubtedly be better health. What's more, a reduction in the severity and frequency of migraines is likely.

Fish oils can be added to the diet simply by eating fish rich in these oils. Fish containing the highest amount of EPA/DHA are cold water fish. This makes sense. Fish living in frigid waters need insulation, and fat serves this function. Those living in the coldest water, such as the Arctic, have the most fatty insulation and, therefore, contain the highest amounts of fish oils. The top sources of fatty fish oils include:

- mackerel
- salmon (especially Atlantic)
- trout (especially lake)
- abalone
- tuna (especially albacore)
- whitefish
- sardines
- herring
- cod
- anchovies
- haddock

Other fish/seafood which contain considerable amounts of fish oils include:

- sablefish
- sturgeon
- bluefish
- shrimp
- crab
- lobster

Migraine patients should eat more of these fish, that is if they are not allergic to them. Ideally, such fish rich in EPA/DHA should be eaten at least twice per week as a means of preventing migraine attacks. The existence of sticky platelets increases the risk for migraine attacks. Such platelets can be normalized, that is their stickiness eliminated, with fish oils. Aspirin or other potentially damaging drugs can also do this, however, their side effects are legion.

Another way to get fish oils is via supplements. EPA/DHA supplements have become popular, particularly in the last decade. They were first introduced by a British company under the trade name *MaxEPA*. Recently, fish oil products have fallen out of vogue as a result of bad publicity. It appears that certain companies, in an effort to get on the bandwagon, have produced and marketed inferior products which have rated poorly when tested and scrutinized by the scientific community. The real scare came when scientists found that some of these products actually caused an increase in cholesterol levels. Further research determined that fish oils, like many oils, have a tendency to become rancid. It is likely that this rancidity caused mild toxicity, and this was manifested by an unexpected rise in cholesterol levels. There is another problem with low-grade fish oil products. Many are made from very large fish; some of these creatures have lived in the oceans for decades. Such fish are more likely to contain high levels of toxic chemicals which can leach into the supplements, since many of these chemicals are fat soluble.

The fact is, recently, it has been shown that the regular intake of fatty fish can poison the individual, that is through heavy metal poisoning. Thus, it may be necessary to modify the intake of such fish, plus once a week or less, eating instead large amounts of smaller fish such as sardines, herring, and anchovies, which are relatively low in heavy metals.

It has been known for years that certain oils, notably the polyunsaturates, easily become rancid, especially if they are heated. The only thing that stops the rancidity is to add preservatives. This is why commercial manufacturers, after producing refined vegetable oils, commonly add the synthetic antioxidants *BHT* and *BHA*. These potent antioxidants prevent the oils from turning rancid during storage, helping prolong shelf life. Unfortunately, these preservatives may themselves be toxic and would be inappropriate for adding to a "health food" supplement. Rather, we must turn to natural antioxidants and preservatives such as garlic, oil of oregano, oil of rosemary, oil of sage, and vitamin E.

Rancid oils are unfit for human consumption. Such oils cause digestive upset, aggravate existing illnesses or may even cause disease. How can you tell if a fish oil product is rancid?

Simply by the smell. The more fishy the odor is, the more rancid it will be. Prolonged aftertaste may also be an indication of rancidity. However, don't let this scare you from using fish oils. People freely use aspirin as a blood thinner. Fish oils are certainly far safer than such dangerous drugs.

Essential Fatty Acids: Migraine Fighters

Essential fatty acids are vegetable oils critical for various organ functions. These fatty acids are known as linoleic and linolenic acids. Without them cells become dysfunctional and in the extreme, die. In contrast, fish oils have not, as of yet, been classified as essential. An essential fatty acid is one which is, as the name implies, essential to life itself. This means that without them human life would fail to exist. Disease and death can result from a prolonged deficiency. This is largely because essential fatty acids must be obtained from the diet and cannot be made within the human body.

Most Americans are deficient in this crucial nutrient. One reason is that we are simply not getting enough of it in the diet. Another is that many commonly consumed substances destroy or block the utilization of essential fatty acids, particularly a unique compound known as *gamma linolenic acid* (GLA). A list of substances and conditions which negatively affect GLA includes:

- birth control pills
- alcohol
- cigarette smoke
- chewing tobacco
- chlorinated water
- deep fried foods
- junk foods
- radiation
- toxic chemicals
- yeast infections
- diabetes
- arthritis
- cancer
- chronic viral illness
- partially hydrogenated or hydrogenated oils

In addition, zinc and B-6 deficiency make it virtually impossible for the body to utilize essential fatty acids; over 60% of Americans are deficient in both zinc and B-6. Symptoms of essential fatty acid/GLA deficiency include dry skin, eczema, brittle or dry hair, hair loss, easy bruising, delayed growth, brittle nails, excessive thirst, increased susceptibility to infection, infertility, dry mouth and/or eyes, thick saliva, delayed wound healing, PMS, dryness and flaking behind the ears, dry patches on the face, greasy skin, greasy hair, prostate disorders, ovarian cysts, and fibrocystic breasts. It is obvious that a lack of essential fatty acids greatly disrupts body functions, with, seemingly, an emphasis upon damage to the endocrine glands.

What does all this have to do with headaches? Remember, the brain is made up primarily of fats which occur biochemically in the form of fatty acids. Among the most important fatty acids in brain function are the ones in which Americans are most commonly deficient—the omega-6 fatty acids, which includes GLA and fish oils, as well as lecithin.

Essential fatty acids are readily absorbed into the brain. This is particularly true of the omega-6's. Such oils help stabilize the nerves, making them less susceptible to disease and inflammation. It has another powerful effect unrelated to the brain. It helps diminish PMS, reducing the occurrence of PMS-induced headaches. GLA, as well as a high quality essential fatty acid oil, should form a part of the anti-migraine nutritional regimen, especially in the case of menstruating women. A dose of 6 to 12 capsules per day of GLA should be sufficient. For an essential fatty acid oil crude fortified pumpkinseed oil, that is the Pumpkinol, is ideal. Crude pumpkinseed oil is rich in both types of essential fatty acids, the linoleic and linolenic acids. It is low in GLA but supplements components which potentiate it. What's more, regarding the Pumpkinol it is a rich source of naturally occurring vitamin E, as well as natural chlorophyll and phytosterols, all of which help regulate cell metabolism. The vitamin E content of Pumpkinol is significant. Three tablespoons provides well over 30 I. U., some two times the RDA. The vitamin E is a complex, not a mere isolate. This makes it significantly more powerful than the commercial type. In fact, 30 I.U. of the crude extract is equal in therapeutic power to some 300 I.U. or more of the isolate. Thus, for reversing hormonal disorders, such as ovarian cysts, uterine disorders, migraines, infertility, and prostate disorders, it is more effective than vitamin E pills. Pumpkinol may be ordered from finer health food stores or by calling 1-800-243-5242.

There is a benefit of the Pumpkinol over the GLA. This is due to the methods of extraction. With GLA solvents are used. Thus, any supplement may contain residues of such chemicals. With Pumpkinol it is strictly a pressed oil, extracted at a slightly raised temperature: a mere 90 degrees Fahrenheit. Thus, it is truly a natural unprocessed extract. This is why it is so rich in naturally occurring nutrients—vitamin E, vitamin K, coenzyme Q-10, chlorophyll, and more.

Conclusion

Migraines, as well as other types of headaches, can be cured. Thus, it is possible to live without headache pain. Using natural medicines, as well as dietary change, can be curative. Usually, migraines can be eliminated by determining the cause and treating it. There is no reason to suffer permanently.

Migraines due to food allergies are the easiest to cure. All that is necessary is to determine what the allergies are and avoid them. Thus, there is no need to suffer forever. If the toxic foods are eliminated, an improvement must occur.

Reactions to foods are the main cause of headaches. There is no one universal list of migraine/headache-provoking foods. Each person's food list will vary. However, cheeses, wine, pork, cocoa, corn, shrimp, wheat, eggs, and coffee are commonly implicated. Yet, virtually any food or food additive can be the culprit. This is why food intolerance testing is recommended. In addition, every person with allergic migraines has a different pattern regarding the type of headache he/she has. Some get headaches immediately after eating the offending food, while in others the headaches occur days after the incident. The pain may last anywhere from a few hours to as long as a week. This pain can occur in multiple regions, in the face, forehead, over the sinuses, behind the eye, along the temple, or back of the head.

Incredibly, there are people who have daily headaches. These headaches can persist for weeks or even months and are often entirely the result of consuming allergenic foods.

This book is a tool to solve the headache dilemma. The goal is to eliminate headaches. This is accomplished through dramatic changes in the diet, including the elimination of allergenic foods. It is also achieved through the aggressive use of nutritional supplements as well as herbal medicines.

A great deal can be accomplished through curing headaches. As a result, a person's entire life can be changed. A life of pain becomes one of pleasure. Sick leave is decreased, productivity is enhanced, and vitality is improved. Overall health is greatly enhanced. What's more, the individual becomes more energetic, not to mention the improved mental outlook and a happier personality which results from excellent health. Eliminating this paralyzing illness lifts a phenomenal burden. Finally, life becomes a pleasurable experience. The burden—the agony—is finally relieved.

There is no need for headache patients to resign themselves to "living with the pain." Some so-called experts in the field would have it believed that headaches are largely incurable. On the contrary, many measures can be taken. This book lists proven remedies. It provides other options, which have been found to be valuable in a clinical setting.

Numerous scientific articles supporting the claims in this book are listed. The migraine patient should at a minimum know one thing: *Migraines have a cause, and a cure is likely to result if that cause is found and effectively treated.* If nothing else, remember this: investigate anything with potential. People take this attitude in other areas of life, including business, sports and pleasure. Why not with health?

It is true that besides allergic reactions there are many other causes of headaches. The list includes infection, hormonal disturbances, chemical sensitivity, muscle tension, high blood pressure, hypothyroidism, adrenal gland disorders, and the more serious conditions such as abscesses and brain tumors. Life-threatening causes of migraines account for a relatively small percentage of cases.

In their desperation most people resort to the use of chemicals and drugs, which act only to treat the symptoms of headaches. Drugs never treat the cause. The list of drugs commonly used for headaches includes aspirin, Bufferin, Excedrin, Motrin, Tylenol, Aleve, Imigran, Zomig, Cafergot, Midrin, Empirin, Valium, Xanax, and Inderal. Some people take drugs—aspirin for example—like they are eating candy and think nothing of it. They should realize the risks of permanent damage to human tissues. Plus, drugs may increase the susceptibility to migraines via the physiological damage they perpetrate. Drugs destroy the lining of the intestines, while contaminating the internal organs. Thus, by disrupting organ function they aggravate the condition.

Drugs do kill pain. If they are eliminated, what remains for controlling the pain? There are few magic pills in nutrition. Enzymes may help. Pantothenic acid boosts the cortisone response. Spice extracts contain potent pain-killing substances. Migraten contains a variety of pain-killing herbs and spices. Two of its components, the P73 wild oregano, and the oil of wild rosemary, have morphine-like actions. What's more, oil of oregano is a potent pain-killer. When taken under the tongue it helps eliminate headaches.

In modern medicine only the symptoms are treated. By neglecting the cause the illness is often prolonged. Thus, the potential for physiological damage is increased. The sooner the problem is diagnosed and corrected, the better off the patient will be. Drug dependency, whether due to narcotics or over-the-counter painkillers, is a dire situation, the negative effects being both physical and mental. Getting off the drugs is an important step in the migraine cure process.

Good nutrition and prevention through food allergy removal can produce spectacular results. A person could be cured of migraines just by avoiding certain foods. Because of this approach, people who have had migraines for decades and who have searched all over this nation are now living free of pain.

In the United States alone twenty five million people have migraines. As many as 60 million Americans have experienced a headache of some sort. That's nearly one fourth of the population. People of fame, past and present, have suffered the illness. They include St. Gregory, Chopin, Charles Darwin, Sigmund Freud, Thomas Jefferson and George Bernard Shaw. Mr. Shaw, the noted British historian, a witty character, confronted another migraine sufferer, the renowned Norwegian North Pole explorer, Fridjof Nansen. He said, "Mr. Nansen, have you found a cure for headaches?" Mr. Nansen replied, "No." Then Mr. Shaw said, "Astonishing . . . you have spent your life trying to discover the North Pole, which nobody cares about, and you have never attempted to discover a cure for headaches which every living person is crying aloud for?" Mr. Shaw and many other famous individuals probably searched in vain for a relief or a cure. Ironically, the cure was more obvious and simple than any of these brilliant men could comprehend.

One need not search the far reaches of the globe for a migraine cure. There is no need to make a valiant effort to glean through the years of accumulated medical research in order to search for some missing link. The cure is within reach: it is what we put in our mouths that causes the vast majority of migraines. Whether that be a cigarette, medicine, alcoholic beverage, coffee or food, this is where it all begins.

It has been said that the origin of illness is largely a consequence of how much people abuse their bodies. The most common abuses involve dietary habits or, more descriptively, habits which control what goes into our bodies. Eating to an excess is one form of abuse. Consuming substances with known toxicity, such as cigarette smoke, alcoholic beverages, and heavily processed foods, are other forms. There is a third abuse, one which is entirely unintentional and one which is difficult to explain. It is the consumption of allergenic foods, which, under any other circumstances, would be good for the body. Is eating broccoli or carrots bad for you? It can be, but *only if you are allergic to them.*

Headaches are second only to colds as the most common complaint in doctors' offices. Tens of billions of dollars are spent each year in attempt to alleviate headache pain. A great deal of this is spent in futility, since the majority of therapies do little more than camouflage the pain. Why wouldn't a person accept a trial of medicine when he/she is told, "It's only nerves" or "You're under too much stress." Fortunately, however, money and time can be spent more judiciously, with better results, permanent cure and less strain over the long haul.

John Mansfield, M.D., British pioneer of allergy research, states in the conclusion of his book, *Migraine and the Allergy Connection*, "Food allergy plays the greatest single part in the causation of this (migraine) disease." Mansfield is one of many modern researchers convinced that migraines are due to food allergies and that proper diagnosis and treatment will lead to a cure.

The alternative treatments for migraine need not be bizarre or unscientific. Nutritional support makes sense and does help. Toxic foods must be removed. Chemicals which poison the body must be cleansed. Certain natural supplements, particularly concentrated herb and spice extracts, provide relief and speed the cure. Any treatment should be based on a sound, scientific, and clinical model. The prescribed treatment methods in this book are scientific and also effective. The focus should be on the appropriate herbal medicines and dietary changes. These solutions will help eliminate this epidemic once and for all. Thus, the individual will finally become pain-free. This is the result of using the powers of nature—created by the authority of the highest being, who brought such cures to the human race. They are available for human beings to take advantage of: to use to regain health. Take advantage of the powers of natural cures. Determine any food allergies, and change the diet. Eliminate the intake of processed foods. Correct any hormonal and/or structural imbalances. Correct any nutritional and/or dietary imbalances. As a result the individual will surely be pain-free.

Appendix A

Foods Containing WHEAT:

beer
biscuits
bouillon cubes
bread: corn, gluten, graham, oat,
   pumpernickel, white, rye, soy
cake
candy
candy bars
cereals
chocolate
cookies
crackers
doughnuts
flour
gin
gravies
ice cream cones
macaroni
matzos
mayonnaise
muffins
noodles
Ovaltine
pancakes, waffles
pizza
pies
popovers
Postum
pretzels
puddings
rolls
sausage, cold meats
synthetic pepper
whiskeys
yeast

Foods Containing EGGS:

baking powders
Bavarian cream
bouillon
breads, breaded foods
cakes
candies
malted cocoa drinks
marshmallows
mayonnaise
meat loaf
meringues
noodles

consommés
cookies
creamed pies
croquettes
custards
doughnuts
French toast
fritters
frostings
Hollandaise sauce
ice cream
icings
macaroni
macaroons
omelets
pancakes
pasta
pretzels
puddings
salad dressing
sausage
sherbet
souffles
soups
tartar sauce
timbales
waffles
wine

Foods Containing SOY BEAN:

bread
cake
candies
cereal
cheese (processed)
cold cuts
flour
fried foods (home and commercial)
gravies
Hamburger Helper
hamburger patties
ice cream
iced milk
margarine
mayonnaise
milk substitutes
nondairy products
nuts
packaged mixes
pastas
pastries
potato chips
rolls
salad dressing
sausage
sherbet
shortenings (liquid/ solid)
soy sauce
vegetable oil
wieners

Foods containing MILK:

au gratin foods
baking powder
Bavarian cream
biscuits
bisques
bologna
bread
breakfast or diet drinks
butter
buttermilk
butter sauces
cakes
candy
chocolate drinks
chowders
cookies
cream cheese
doughnuts
eggs (scrambled)
flour mixtures: biscuit,
    muffin, cake, waffle,
    pancake, pudding
gravies
hot cakes
ice cream
mashed potatoes
malted milk
meat loaf
omelet
popovers
protein powders
salad dressings
sherbet
soda crackers
souffles
soup

Foods Containing PORK:

bacon
bacon drippings
bakery products
candy bars
canned meat
Chinese food
chitterlings (chitlings)
gelatin, Jello etc.
ham
ice cream (mono/diglycerides)
lard
pancake mixes
pickled pigs feet
Polynesian food
pork and beans
pork rinds
potato chips
Fritos etc
pre-breaded frozen foods,
    (frozen seafood/fish).
puddings
salad dressings

liverwurst
lunch meat
margarine
mashed potatoes (instant)
mayonnaise
Mexican food (tortillas etc.)
mincemeat
non-dairy cream, Coffee Mate, etc.

salads
sausage
shortening
Spam
vegetable stock
Vienna sausage
wieners

Foods Containing YEAST:

bacon
barbecue sauce
bread
buns
butter
cake and cake mix
canned fruit and vegetables
cheese (all kinds)
chili peppers
condiments
cookies
crackers
flour enriched with vitamins
    from yeast
French dressing
frozen or canned citrus fruit juices
Gerber's oatmeal
ham
horseradish
jam
jelly
ketchup

milk fortified with
    vitamins from yeast
mince pie
molasses
mushrooms
olives
pastries
pickles
preserves
pretzels
rolls, homemade and
    canned
root beer
salad dressing
sauerkraut
sour cream
syrup
tomato sauce
truffles
vitamin tablets/capsules
vinegar (apple, pear,
    grape and distilled)

malted products (cereal, candy,
malted milk drinks)
mayonnaise
meat fried in cracker crumbs

alcohol (whiskey, wine,
brandy, rum, vodka,
beer and gin)

Foods Containing COTTONSEED OIL:

breaded frozen foods
breads, rolls and buns
cake, cookie and pastry mixes
candies
deep fried foods
foods processed by commercial frying and baking, doughnuts
frozen pizza
lard or solid shortening
margarine
mayonnaise
microwave popcorn
pastries, pies and cakes
salad oils
sardines (may be packed in cottonseed oil)
snack foods of all types (chips, crackers, cookies)

Sources of Added NITRATES in Food:

bacon
bologna
bratwurst
chipped beef
corn dogs
corned beef
ham
head cheese
hot dogs

pork and beans
salami
sausage
sliced chicken and
turkey breast (some)
smoked salmon (and
other smoked fish)
smoked turkey
Spam

jerky

liverwurst

pickled pigs feet

pastrami

turkey bologna

turkey ham

turkey salami

Note: Even if a person is not allergic to nitrates or the foods containing them, it is possible to get a headache due to the nitrate-induced chemical toxicity of the blood.

Foods containing SULFITES:

baked goods

batters

breadings

canned fruits

canned vegetables

coffee

cole slaw

cornstarch

dried fruits

fish products (including fresh fish)

frozen vegetables

fruit drinks

fruit salad

fruit toppings

gelatins

gravies and sauces

guacamole

hard candy

instant tea

jams and jellies

jarred fruits

olives

pancake syrup

pickles

pie fillings

potato chips

potato salad

puddings

relishes

salad dressings

soups (canned or dried)

tortilla chips

vinegars

white and brown sugar

Foods Containing MSG:

Accent or Lawry's seasoning

bacon bits

baking mixes

batters
beef jerky
bouillon cubes
bread stuffings
breaded, deep fried foods
breaded/frozen foods
breadings
brown or creamy gravies and sauces
canned meats
canned tuna (Chicken of the Sea, Bumble Bee, and Geisha brands)
cheese dips and sauces
cheese puffs
Chef Boyardee products
chicken and beef spreads
chili, canned (Hormel)
Chinese food, canned
chip dip
clam chowder
corn or tortilla chips
croutons
dry roasted nuts (Planters)
frozen dinners (Swanson's, Morton, Weight Watchers, Lean Cuisine)
frozen pizza
frozen pot pies
frozen potato products (French fries, Tater Tots)
gelatins
packed noodles or pasta
potato chips
processed and cured meats (hot dogs, bologna, bacon, etc.)
processed cheeses
processed poultry products
puddings
relishes

salad dressings
salt substitutes
seasonings
soft candies
soups, canned or dried
soy sauce
stew, canned

Foods Containing SALICYLATES:

almonds
apples
apricots
blackberries
cherries
cloves
cucumbers and pickles
currants
gooseberries
grapes and raisins
mint flavors
nectarines

oranges
peaches
peppermint
raspberries
spearmint
strawberries
tea, all varieties
tomatoes
wines
wine vinegars
wintergreen

APPENDIX B

List of Foods Evaluated for Allergies
Via Food Intolerance Test

Seafood

clam

crab

lobster

oyster

scallop

shrimp

Fish

bass

carp

catfish

caviar

cod

flounder

haddock

halibut

herring

lake perch

lake trout

mackerel

orange roughy

pike

red snapper

salmon

sardine

sea perch

shark

smelt

sole

swordfish

tuna

Poultry

chicken

chicken egg yolk

chicken egg white

duck

pheasant

turkey

Red Meat

beef
lamb
pork

Milk Products

bleu cheese
butter
buttermilk
cheddar cheese
cottage cheese
cow's milk

goat's milk
mozzarella cheese
Parmesan cheese
provolone cheese
Swiss cheese
yogurt

Grains

barley
millet
oats
rice

rye
wheat
wheat bran

Fruit

apple
apricot
avocado
banana
blackberry
blueberry
cantaloupe
cherry
coconut
date
fig
grape

mango
nectarine
olive
orange
papaya
peach
pear
pineapple
plum (prune)
pomegranate
raspberry
rhubarb

grapefruit
honeydew melon
lemon
lime

strawberry
tomato
watermelon

Vegetables

alfalfa sprouts
artichoke
asparagus
beet
broccoli
Brussels sprouts
cabbage
carrot
cauliflower
celery
chicory
chestnut
corn
cucumber
eggplant
endive
garden (bell) pepper
garlic

green bean
kale
lettuce
okra
onions
parsley
parsnip
pimento
pumpkin
radish
rutabagas
spinach
squash
string beans
Swiss chard
turnip
watercress
water chestnuts

Nuts and Seeds

almond
black walnut
Brazil nut
cashew
chestnuts
English walnut

filbert
pecan
pistachio
safflower seed (oil)
sesame seed (oil)
sunflower seed

Spices

allspice
anise seed
basil
bay leaf
black pepper
caraway seed
chili pepper
chives
cinnamon
clove
cumin seed
curry

dill seed
ginger
marjoram
nutmeg
oregano
paprika
peppermint (spearmint)
rosemary
sage
thyme
turmeric

Sweeteners

beet sugar
cane sugar
honey
malt
maple sugar
molasses

NutraSweet
saccharin
sucralose
sorbitol
sorghum

Beans and Legumes

bean sprouts
black-eyed peas
carob
chick pea
kidney beans
lentil

lima bean
mung bean
peanut
pinto bean
soybean
split pea

Miscellaneous

baker's yeast
brewer's yeast
cocoa
coffee
cola
cottonseed oil
food dyes
frog legs
gelatin
hops
MSG

mushroom
potato
salicylate
sulfites
sweet potato
tapioca
tea
tobacco
vanilla
yam

Appendix C

Physicians, Laboratories, and Supplements

The following is a list of physicians skilled at performing allergy testing as described in this book for diagnosing allergy-induced migraine:

Better Health Center
Dr. Bob Martin
5727 N. 7th Street,
Suite 300
Phoenix, Arizona 85014
(602) 266-7246

Menner Chiropractic
165 South Rand Road
Lake Zurich, Illinois 60047
(847) 540-6060

Optimum Health Center
850 Marsh Street, Suite C
Valparaiso, Indiana 46385
(219) 462-3377

Middlebury Chiropractic Clinic
Norman Miller, D.O.
516 S. Main Street
Middlebury, Indiana 46540
(219) 825-9124

Dr. Susan Player
519 Cleveland, Suite #211
Clearwater, Florida 34615
(813) 449-0121

Richard Hrdlicka, MD
302 Randall
Geneva, Illinois 60134
(708) 232-1900

Laboratories

Leaky Gut Syndrome,
Secretory IgA

Diagnos-Techs
6620 S. 192nd Place
Building J
Kent, Washington 98032
(800) 878-3787

Hair Analysis,
Toxic Metal Screen

Doctor's Data
3755 Illinois Avenue
St. Charles, Illinois 60174-2420
(800) 323-2784

Nutritional Supplements
(mentioned in this book)

See: wildoreganoonline.com
oreganol.com
or call: 1-800-243-5242

Bibliography

Abraham, G.E. and M.M. Lubran. 1981. Serum and red cell magnesium levels in patients with premenstrual tension. *American Journal of Clinical Nutrition.* 34:23642366.

Anderson, R.A., Bryden, N.A., et al. 1985. Chromium supplementation of human subjects. *Nutrition Research,* suppl.1: 56063.

Ammann, A.J., and R. Long. 1970. Selective IgA deficiency and autoimmunity. *Clin. Exp. Immunol.* 7:83338.

Ammann, A.J., and R. Long. 1971. Selective IgA deficiency: representation of 30 cases and a review of the literature. *Medicine* 50:22336.

Arora, R.B., et al. 1971. Anti-inflammatory studies on curcuma longa (turmeric). *Ind. J. Med. Res.* 59(8):1289.

Bali, L. 1978. Vitamin C and migraine: a case report. *N.E.J.M.* (letter to the editor) Aug. 17, p. 364.

Barnes, B.O., and C.W. Barnes. 1972. *Heart Attack Rareness in Thyroid Treated Patients.* Charles C. Thomas, Springfield, Ill.

Barnes, B.O., and L. Galton. 1976. *Hypothyroidism: The Unsuspected Illness.* Thomas Y. Crowell Co., New York.

Bernstein, I.D., et al. 1968. Absorption of antigens from the gastrointestinal tract. *Int. Arch. Allergy Applied Immuno.* 33:52129.

Bille, B.1962. Migraine in school children. *Acta Paediat.* suppl.51:136.

Bjarnason, I., Ward, K., et al. 1984. The leaky gut of alcoholism: possible route of entry for toxic compounds. *Lancet* 28, Jan.

Bjarnason, I., et al. 1984. Intestinal permeability and inflammation in rheumatoid arthritis: effects of nonsteroidal anti-inflammatory drugs. *Lancet* Nov. 24, p. 42.

Bjarnason, I., et al. 1987. Blood and protein loss via small intestinal inflammation induced by nonsteroidal anti-inflammatory drugs. *Lancet* 2:711–715.

Blau, J.N. 1984. Towards a definition of migraine headache. *Lancet* I : 44445.

Bock, S.A., and C.D. May. 1983. Adverse reactions to food caused by sensitivity. In Middleton, E., Jr., Reed, C.E., and Ellis, E.F., eds.: *Allergy Principles and Practice.* C.V. Mosby Co. St. Louis, Mo. pp. 1415-25.

Bogduk, N. 1980. The anatomy of occipital neuralgia. *Clin. Exp. Neuro.* 17:167.

Bourcher, R.C., Pare, P.D., and J.C. Hogg. 1979. Relationship between airway hyperactivity and hyperpermeability in ascaris sensitive monkeys. *J. Allergy Clin. Immunol.* 64:197-201.

Breneman, J.C. 1978. *Basics of Food Allergy.* Charles C. Thomas, Springfield, Ill.

Bryan, W.T.K., and M.P. Bryan. 1971. Cytotoxic reaction in the diagnosis of food allergy. *Otolaryngol. Clin. N. Am.* 4:523-34.

Buckley, R.H., et al. 1969. Correlation of milk precipitins with IgA deficiency. *N.E.J.M.* 281:465-69.

Buist, R. 1984. *Food Intolerance: What It Is and How to Cope With It.* Harper & Rowe, Sydney, Australia.

Busse, W.W., Koop, D.E., and E. Middleton. 1984. Flavonoid modulation of human neutrophil function. *J. Allergy Clin. Immunol.* 73:801-9.

Caradoc-Davies, T.H. 1984. Nonsteroidal anti-inflammatory drugs, arthritis, and gastrointestional bleeding in elderly inpatients. *Age and Aging* 13:295-98.

Clark, D. 1948. The endocrine approach to the treatment of allergy. *Ann. Western Med. Surg.* 22(9):404-407.

Clausen, J. 1988. Chromium induced clinical improvement in symptomatic hypoglycemia. *Bio. 71 Elem. Res.* 17:229-36.

Congon, P.J., and W.l. Forsythe. 1979. Migraine and childhood; a study of 300 children. *Develop. Med. Child. Neurol.* 21:209-16.

Couch, J.R., and R.S. Hassenein. 1977. Platelet aggregability in migraine. *Neurology* 27:643.

Cousins, N.1979. *Anatomy of an Illness.* W.W. Norton & Co., New York.Crabbe', P.A., Carbonaro, A.O., and J.F. Heremans. 1965. The normal human intestinal mucosa as a major source of plasma cells containing IgA. *Int. Acad. Path.* 14(3):23539.

Crabbe', P.A., Bazin, H., Eyssen, H., et al. 1968. The normal flora as a major stimulus for proliferation of plasma cells synthesizing IgA in the gut. *Int. Arch. Allergy* 34:36275.

Crayton, J.W., Stone, T., and G.G. Stein. 1981. Epilepsy precipitated by food sensitivity: report of a case with double-blind placebo controlled assessment. *Clin. Electroencephalogr.* 12(4): 1928.

D'Anglejan-Chatillon, J., et al. 1989. Migraine—a risk factor for dissection of cervical arteries. *J.A.M.A.* Vol. 263 No. 17.

Dalton, K. 1975. Food intake prior to a migraine attack: study of 2,313 spontaneous attacks. *Headache* 15(3): 18893.

Degowin, E.L. 1932. Allergic migraine: a review of sixty cases. *J. Allergy* 3:55766.

Delespesse, G., et al. 1976. Cellular aspect of selective IgA deficiency. *Clin. Exp. Immunol.* 24:27379.

Deluca, L.M., et al. 1986. Vitamin A and the liver. *Prog. Liver Dis.* 8:8198.

Diamond, S.D. 1988. *Hope for your Headache Problem.* Revised ed. International Univ. Press, Madison.

Donovan, E.W. 1985. *Essentials of Pathophysiology.* Macmillan Publishing Co., New York.

Drummond, P.D., and J.W. Lance. 1983. Extracranial vascular changes and the source of pain in migraine headache. *Ann. Neuro.* 13:32.

Eaton, C.D. 1954. Co-existence of hypothyroidism with diabetes mellitus. *J. Mich. Med. Soc.* 53:1101.

Egger, J., Carter, C.M., Wilson, J., et al. 1983. Is migraine food allergy? A double blind controlled trial of oligoantigenic diet treatment. *Lancet* 2:865868.

Egger, J., Carter, M., Soothill, J.F., et al. 1989. Oligoantigenic diet treatment of children with epilepsy and migraine. J. *Pediatrics* 114(1):5157.

Ensminger, A.H., et al. 1983. *Foods and Nutrition Encyclopedia.* Vol. 1&2, Pergus Press, Clovis, CA.

Eyermann, C.H. 1931. Allergic headache. J. *Allergy* 2:106-12.

Ferrari, A., and E. Sternieri. 1990. Dietary headaches through the centuries. *Funct. Neurol.* 5:79-84.

Fredericks, C., and H. Goodman. 1969. *Low Blood Sugar and You.* Constellations International, New York.

Freed, D.L.F. 1978. Mucotractive effect of lectin. *Lancet* 1:585-6.

Freed, D.L.F., and R.J. Cooper. 1977. Cytotoxicity of bread and soya protein in tissue culture. *Lancet* 2:371.

Giacovazzo, M., and P. Martelletti. 1989. Letter to the editor. *Ann. Allergy* 63:255.

Glover, V., Snadler, M., Grant, E., et al. 1977. Transitory decrease in platelet monoamine oxidase activity during migraine attacks. *Lancet* 1:391-93.

Gold, M. 1982. Significant number of depressives may have hypothyroidism. *Family Practice News* Nov. 1.

Goltman, M.A. 1936. Mechanism of migraine. J. *Allergy* 7:351.

Gotze, H. 1975. Enteropancreatic circulation of digestive enzymes as a conservation mechanism. *Nature* 257:60-79.

Graham, J.R., and H.G. Wolff. 1937. Mechanisms of migraine headache and action of ergotamine tartrate. *Illinois Med. J.* 99:210.

Grant, E.G. 1965. Relation of arterioles in the endometrium to headache from oral contraceptives. *Lancet* 1:1 143-44.

Grant, E.G., Albuquerque, M., Steiner, T.J., et al. 1978. Oral contraceptives, smoking and ergotamine in migraine. *Current Concepts in Migraine Research.* R. Greene, ed. Raven Press, New York.

Grant, E.G. 1979. Food allergies and migraine. *Lancet* 1:966-69.

Gunn, C.C., and W.E. Milbrandt. 1977. Utilizing trigger points. *Osteopathic Physician* Mar.

Hanington, E. 1971. Migraine. *Trans. Med. Soc.* 87:32.

Hanington, E., Jones, R.J., Arness, J.A., et al. 1981. Migraine: a platelet disorder. *Lancet* 2:720-23.

Harrison, D.P. 1986. Copper as a factor in the dietary precipitation of migraine. *Headache* 26(5):248-50.

Havsteen, B. 1983. Flavonoids, a class of natural products of high pharmacological potency. *Biochem. Pharm.* 32: 1121-8.

Heaney, R.P., and R.R. Recker. 1986. Distribution of calcium absorption in middle aged women. *Am. J. Clin. Nutr.* 43:229-305.

Heatley, R.V., Denburg, J.A., Bayer, N., et al. 1982. Increased plasma histamine levels in migraine patients. *Clin. Allergy* 12:145-49.

Henderson, W.R., and N.H. Raskin. 1972. Hotdog headache: individual susceptibility to nitrite. *Lancet* 2:1162.

Hollander, D., and H. Tarnawski. 1985. Aging associated increase in intestinal absorption of macromolecules. *Gerontology* 31:133-137.

Horrobin, D. F. 1981. The importance of gamma-linolenic acid and prostaglandin El in human nutrition and medicine. *J. Holistic Med.* 3(2): 11839.

Hurxthal, L.M. 1934. Blood cholesterol and thyroid disease. *Arch. Int. Med.* 53:825.

Jameson, S., Arfors, K., et al. 1985. Pain relief and selenium balance in patients with connective tissue disease and osteoarthrosis: a double blind selenium tocopherol supplementation study. *Nutrition Research* suppl. 1:391-397.

Jennings, I.W. 1970. *Vitamins in Endocrine Metabolism.* Charles C. Thomas, Springfield, Ill.

Johns, D.R.1986. Migraine provoked by aspartame. *N.E. J.M.* 315:456.

Kabacoff, B.L., et al. 1963. Absorption of chymotryspin from the intestinal tract. *Nature* 199:815.

Kailin, E.W., and A. Hastings. 1966. Electromyographic evidence of DDT-induced myoasthenia. *Medical Annals District Columbia* 35:237.

Kailin, E.W., and A. Hastings. 1970. Electromyographic evidence of cerebral malfunction in migraine due to egg allergy. *Medical Annals District Columbia* 39(8):437-41.

Koehler, S., and A. Glaros. 1988. The effect of aspartame on migraine headache. *Headache* 28: 10 13.

Kohlenberg, R.J. 1982. Tyramine sensitivity in dietary migraine: a critical review. *Headache* 22:30-4.

Kountz, W.B. 1951. *Thyroid Function and its Possible Role in Vascular Degeneration.* Charles C. Thomas, Springfield, Ill.

Lake-Bakaar, G., et al. 1982. Origin of circulating serum immunoreactive trypsin in man. *Dig Dis. Sci.* 27(2):143-48.

Langer, S.E., and J.F. Scheer. 1984. *Solved: The Riddle of Illness.* Keats Publishing, Inc., New Canaan, Conn.

Lessof, M.H., Wraith, D.G., Merrett, T.G., et al. 1980. Food allergy and intolerance in 100 patients—local and systemic effects. *Q.J. Med.* 49:259-71.

Lessof, M.H. (ed). 1983. *Clinical Reactions to Foods.* John Wiley & Sons, Chichester.

Lewit, K.1979. Needle effect in relief of myofascial pain. *Pain* 6:8390.

Liener, I.E. (ed). 1969. *Toxic Constituents of Plant Foodstuffs.* Academic Press, New York.

Lipton, R., Newman, L., Cohen, J., et al. 1989. Aspartame as a dietary trigger of headache. Headache 29:90-2.

Littlewood, J., Glover, V., and M. Sandler. 1982. Platelet

Liu, V.J.K., and R.P. Abernathy. 1982. Chromium and insulin in young subjects with normal glucose tolerance. *Am. J. Clin. Nutr.* 35:6617.

Livingston, J.N., and B.J. Purvis. 1980. Effects of wheat germ agglutinin on insulin binding and insulin sensitivity of fat cells. *Am. J. Physiol.* 238:267-75.

Maher, T., and R. Wurtman. 1987. Possible neurologic effects of aspartame, a widely used food additive. *Envir. H. Per.* 75:53-7.

Makuta, M., et al. 1986. Application of eicosapentaenoic acid to health food. *Jpn. Sudo. Saiensu* 25(1):29-35.

Male, D., and I.M. Roitt. 1979. Analysis of the components of immune complexes. *Mol. Immunol.* 16:197.

Manington, E., Horn, M., and M. Wilkinson, eds. 1970. In: Cochrane, A.L., ed. *Third Migraine Symposium* 1969. Heinemann, London.

Mansfield, J. 1990. *Migraine and the Allergy Connection.* Healing Arts Press, Rochester, Vermont.

Mansfield, L.E., Vaughan, T.R., Waller, S.F., et al. 1985. Food allergy and adult migraine: double-blind and mediator confirmation of an allergic etiology. *Ann. Allergy* 55:126-29.

Mansfield, L.E. 1987. The role of food allergy in migraine: a review. *Ann. Allergy* 58:313-16.

Mansfield, L.E. 1988. Food allergy and headache. *Postgraduate Medicine* 83(7):46-55.

Martinez, O.B., MacDonald, A.C., et al. 1985. Dietary chromium and effect of chromium supplementation on glucose tolerance of elderly Canadian women. *Nutrition Research* 5:609-20.

May, C.D., and S.A. Block. 1978. A modern clinical approach to food hypersensitivity. *Allergy* 33:166.

Medina, J., and S. Diamond. 1978. The role of diet in migraine. *Headache* 18(1):31-4.

Melzack, R. 1981. Myofascial trigger points: relation to acupuncture and mechanism of pain. *Arch. Phys. Med. Rehabil.* May, Vol. 62 (symposium).

Merrett, J., Peatsfield, R.C., Clifford Rose, F., et al. 1983. Food related antibodies in headache patients. *J. Neurol. Neurosurg Psych.* 46:738-42.

Middleton, E. 1984. The flavonoids, trends in pharmaceutical science. *Science* 5:335-8.

Mike, N., Haeney, M.R., Goodwin, B.J.F., et al. 1983. Soya protein antibodies in man: their occurrence and possible relevance in coeliac disease. In: *The Second Fisons Food Allergy Workshop.* Medicine Publishing Foundation, Oxford.

Moffett, A.M., Swash, M., and D.F. Scott. 1974. Effect of chocolate in migraine: a double blind study. *J. Neurol. Neurosurg. Psych.* 37:445-8.

Moncada, S., et al. 1986. Leucocytes and tissue injury: The use of eicosapentaenoic acid in the control of white cell activation. *Wien. Klin. Wochenschr.* 98(4):104-06.

Monro, J., Brostoff, J., Carini, C., et al. 1980. Food allergy in migraine: study of dietary exclusion and RAST. *Lancet* 2:1-4.

Monro, J., Carini, C., and J. Brostoff. 1984. Migraine is a food-allergic disease. *Lancet* 2:719-21.

Monte, W.C. 1984. Aspartame: Methanol and the public health. *J. Appl. Nutr.* 36:42-53.

Morley, J.E. 1982. Food Peptides—a new class of hormones? *J.A.M.A.* 17:2379-80.

Nicklas, R.A. 1989. Sulfites: A review with emphasis on biochemistry and clinical application. *Allergy Proc.* 10(5):349-55.

Noah, N.D., et al. 1980. Food poisoning from raw kidney beans. *Br. Med. J.* 2:236-7.

Nylander, M. 1986. Mercury in pituitary glands of dentists. *Lancet* 478:442 Feb.

Oelgoetz, A.W., et al. 1935. The treatment of food allergy and indigestion of pancreatic origin with pancreatic enzymes. *Am. J. Digest. Dis. Nutr.* 2:422-6.

Oelgoetz, A.W., et al. 1936. Further studies in food allergy. *Med. Rec.* 143:20-25.

Oelgoetz, A.W., et al. 1936. Etiology and treatment of food allergy. *Southwestern Med.* 20:463-5.

Oelgoetz, A.W., et al. 1939. Pancreatic enzymes and food allergy. *Med. Rec.* 150:276-9.

Offenbacher, E.G., Rinko, C.J., et al. 1985. The effects of inorganic chromium and brewer's yeast on glucose tolerance, plasma lipids and plasma chromium in elderly subjects. *Am. J. Clin. Nutr.* 42:454-461.

Paganelli, R., Levinsky, R.J., Brostoff, J., et al. 1983. Immune complexes containing food proteins in normal and atopic subjects. *Lancet* 1:1270-72.

Pinckney, E.R. 1983. The accuracy and significance of medical testing. *Arch. Int. Med.* 143(3):512.

Podell, R.N. 1984. Is migraine a manifestation of food allergy? *Postgraduate Med.* 75(4):221-25.

Randolf, T.G., and F. Rawling. 1946. Variations in total leukocytes following test feeding of foods: an appraisal of the individual food test. *Ann. Allergy* 4:163-78.

Randolf, T.G. 1962. *Human Ecology and Susceptibility to the Chemical Environment.* Charles C. Thomas, Springfield, Ill.

Randolf, T.G., Rawling, F., Brostoff, J., et al. 1979. Immune complexes contain food proteins in normal and atopic subjects after oral challenge and effect of sodium cromoglycate on antigen absorption. *Lancet,* pp. 1270-71.

Rapoport, A.M., and F.D. Sheftell. 1990. *Headache Relief:* Simon and Schuster, New York.

Rice, S.L., Eiten Miller, R.R., and P.E. Koehler. 1976. Biologically active amines in food: a review. *J. Milk Food Technol.* 39:353-8.

Rinkel, H.J., Randolf, T.G., and M. Zeller. 1950. *Food Allergy.* Charles C. Thomas, Springfield, Ill.

Rowe, A.H. 1931. *Food Allergy: Its Manifestations, Diagnosis, and Treatment.* Lea & Febiger, Philadelphia.

Rubin, D. 1981. Myofascial trigger point syndromes: an approach to management. *Arch. Phys. Med. Rehabil.* Vol. 62 (symposium) Mar.

Ryan, R.E. 1960. A new approach to the symptomatic treatment of migraine. *Arch. Otolaryng.* 72:325.

Sansum, W.D. 1932. Treatment of indigestion, underweight and allergy with old and new forms of digestive agents. *Southwestern Med.* 16:452-62.

Schwartz, G.R. 1988. *In Bad Taste: The MSG Syndrome.* Signet Books (Penguin Press), New York.

Stevenson, D. 1979. Food allergies and migraine. *Lancet* 14:103.

Stratton, S.A. 1982. Role of endorphins in pain modulation. *J. Ortho. Sports Phys. Ther.* 3(4):200-05.

Swain, A., Dutton, S.P., and A.S. Truswell. 1985. Salicylates in foods. *J. Amer. Diet. Assoc.* 85:950-60.

Taylor, E. 1979. Food additives, allergy and hyperkinesis. *J. Child Psychol. Psychiatry* 20:357-63.

Terano, T., Salmon, J.A., Higgs, G.A., et al. 1986. EPA as a modulator of inflammation: effect upon prostaglandin and leukotriene synthesis. *Biochem. Pharm.* 35(3):779-85.

Todd, L.C. 1933. Food allergy with special reference to migraine. *South. Med. Surg.* pp. 587-92.

Travell, J. 1949. Basis for multiple uses of local block of somatic trigger areas (procaine infiltration and ethylchloride spray). *Mississippi Valley Med. J.* 71:1221.

Travell, J. 1967. Mechanical headache. *Headache* 7:23-29.

Travell, J. 1981. Identification of myofascial trigger point syndrome; a case of atypical facial neuralgia. *Arch. Phys. Med. Rehabil.* V62 (symposium) Mar.

Unger, L., and A.H. Unger. 1951. A new (sublingual) method for controlling the pain of migraine. *Illinois Med. J.* 99:210.

Unger, A.H.1952. Migraine is an allergic disease. *J. Allergy* 23:42940.

Unger, L., and J. Cristol. 1970. Allergic Migraine. *Ann. of Allergy* 28:106-08.

Vahlquist, B. 1955. Migraine in children. *Int. Arch. Allergy Sppl. Immunol.* 7:348-55.

Vaughan, W.T. 1927. Allergic Migraine. *J.A.M.A.* 88:1383-86.

Walker, W.A. 1981. *Intestinal Transport of Macromolecules. Physiology of the Gastrointestinal Tract.* L.R. Johnson, ed., Raven Press, New York.

Walker, W.A. 1982. Mechanisms of antigen handling by the gut. *Clinics Immunol. Allergy.* 2(1): 15-25.

Walzer, A., et al. 1935. Studies in absorption of undigested proteins in human beings; new technique for quantitatively studying absorption and elimination of antigens: preliminary report. *J. Allergy* 6:532-538.

Walzer, M. 1941. Allergy of the abdominal organs. *J. Lab. Clin. Med.* 26:1867.

Warshaw, L., et al. 1971. Small intestinal permeability to macromolecules. *Lab. Invest.* 25:631-39.

Waters, W.E. 1974. *The Epidemiology of Migraine.* Boehringer Ingleheim, Berkshire.

Webber, T.P. 1973. Diagnosis and medication of headache and shoulder-arm-hand syndrome. *J.A.0A.* 72:697-710.

Weeks, V.D., and J. Travell. 1957. How to give painless injections. In *Amer. Med. Assoc.: Scientific Exhibils.*

Weiser, M.M., and A.P. Douglas. 1976. An alternative mechanism for gluten toxicity in coeliac disease. *Lancet* 1:567.

Werner, S.C., and S.H. Ingbar, eds. 1965. *The Thyroid.* Harper & Row, New York.

Whybrow, M.B., et al. 1969. Mental changes accompanying thyroid gland dysfunction. *Archives of General Psychiatry* 20:48.

Wide L., Bennich, H., and S.G.O. Johansson. 1967. Diagnosis of allergy by an invitro test for allergen antibodies. *Lancet* 2:1105.

Wren, J.C. 1968. Thyroid function and coronary atherosclerosis. *J. Amer. Ger. Soc.* 16:696-704.

Wurtman, R.J., and J.J. Wurtman. 1983. Physiological and Behavioral Effects of Food Constituents. *Nutrition and the Brain.* Vol. 6 Raven Press, New York.

Zioudrou, C., and W.A. Klee. 1979. Possible roles of peptides derived from food proteins in brain function. *Nutrition and the Brain.* 4: 12552.

Index

Additional Knowledge House Books

#1 *The Cure is in the Cupboard: How to Use Oregano for Better Health—* $19.95

203 pages–Revised Edition 51/2 x 81/2 inch softback ISBN 0911119744
Oregano helps you regain your health and then stay healthy. This is what saved Dr. Ingram's life. Learn how to use oregano and its essential oil for fighting infection and eliminating pain. Combat skin disorders, injuries, wounds, and dental problems. Particularly valuable for fungal infections.

#2 *Natural Cures For Kiler Germs—*$19.95

342 pages, 6x 9 inch softback ISBN 1931078009
Learn the warning signs of killer germ infections and how you can immunize yourself against them naturally. Learn also the most potent natural cures for reversing colds, flu, sinus disorders, diarrhea, TB, Lyme, hepatitis, blood poisoning, staph infection, candidiasis, West Nile, systemic fungus and vaccine reactions.

#3 *Nutrition Tests For Better Health*—$24.95

330 pages   5 1/2 x 8 1/2 inch softbound   ISBN 193108084
Test yourself to determine your nutritional deficiencies from *A to zinc*. Other tests show evidence of possible health problems such as adrenal insufficiency, chemical toxicity, thyroid insufficiency, intestinal malabsorption, liver dysfunction, and premature aging. Sugar, caffeine, sulfite, food dye, and MSG overload also evaluated. Each test followed by specific and thorough nutritional recommendations. Find out what you are lacking.

#4 *Lifesaving Cures—*$19.95

312 pages, 6x 9 inch softback ISBN 1931078009
To survive in the 21st century you must know lifesaving cures. This book describes the most powerful remedies for reversing everyday illnesses. With this book of natural cures Dr. Ingram provides hundreds of natural answers for dozens of ailments.

#5 *How to Eat Right and Live Longer*—$21.95

373 pages   6 x 9 inch softbound   ISBN 0911119213
Dr. Ingram's most comprehensive book on diet and nutrition. Describes the treatment of a wide range of illnesses through diet and nutritional supplementation. Emphasis is on the nutritional treatment of heart disease, high cholesterol, high triglycerides, diabetes, obesity, allergies, arthritis, neurological disorders, and alcoholism. Step-by-step nutritional protocols, dietary instruction, personalized nutritional/blood analysis, and 100 recipes included.

#6   Supermarket Remedies—$29.95
325 pages   6 1/4 x 9 1/4 inch hardbound   ISBN 0911119647
Reverse health problems with foods, herbs, and spices. Learn to shop for your ailments at the supermarket, health store, and farmer's market. A supermarket juice that reverses heart disease, a vegetable that halts depression, a berry which eliminates stomach aches, a fruit which lowers cholesterol, a berry for poor vision, a protein for great energy, a spice which kills germs and much more. Use supermarket remedies for hundreds of ailments.

#7   The Respiratory Solution—$14.95
206 pages, 5.5x 8.5 inch softback ISBN 1931078076
Learn the most powerful natural cures for reversing dozens of respiratory ailments. Gain fast relief from sinus problems, allergies, mold, bronchial problems, colds, flu and much more using edible natural foods and herbs.

#8   The Longevity Solution—$12.95
144 pages, 5.5x 8.5 inch softback ISBN 1931078017
A book that explains the incredible powers of royal jelly. Reverse fatigue, hormonal problems, hot flashes, anxiety, depression, insomnia, irritability, panic attacks, and much more. Stall the aging process with royal jelly.

Cassette Tapes and Programs

Tape #1   *How to Use Oregano for Common Illnesses—$10.00*

Tape #2   *Professional Series (tapes and manual)—$89.95*

Tape #3   *Wild Oregano, Lifesaving Spice—$10.00*

TO ORDER BOOKS AND CASSETTES:

Make checks payable to: NAHS P.O. Box 4885
Buffalo Grove, IL 60089
telephone: (800) 243-5242

*Shipping Charges: $6.00 for single books—add $1.00 for each additional book. Cassette tape series add $4.00. Payment by check, money order, or credit card.

Use the following for VISA, Mastercard or American Express orders:

Credit Card # _____ Exp. Date _____

Name _____

Address _____

City _____State _____Zip_____